FOR
F**DS
SAKE

What you really need to know about processed food.

From a former food technologist

Min Sheen Tan

For Foods Sake
What you really need to know about processed
food from a former food technologist

First published in Australia by The Food Catalyst Pty Ltd 2026
https://ffoodssake.com/

A catalogue record for this
book is available from the
National Library of Australia

ISBN: 978-1-7644922-0-1 (pbk)
ISBN: 978-1-7644922-1-8 (ebk)

Typesetting and design by Publicious Book Publishing
Published in collaboration with Publicious Book Publishing
www.publicious.com.au

This book is dedicated to my food loving parents
and for those who want to start making a
positive difference in their lives through food.

Contents

Acknowledgements

This first book is the culmination of my years of experience as a food technologist, and it would not have been possible without the support of my former colleagues, friends, mentors, early supporters, and family.

I'm deeply grateful to my parents, Russell and May, for supporting me in writing my first book and always encouraging me to keep going. Your support means more than I can say.

To my former colleagues in the food industry, thank you for your encouragement and for reminding me that this perspective was worth sharing.

I also want to thank the many people I had the privilege of working with across the food industry and for the medical professionals, therapists and coaches who gave me their input. Your dedication, curiosity, and complexity helped shape my understanding of this fascinating world. Every product, every factory floor conversation, and every quality control challenge added depth to this book.

I'm especially thankful to my editor, Judith Huang, and to the designers (Luyuan Yang and Sarah Lim), and the publishing team who helped bring this project to life. Your care, talent, and patience helped shape it into its final form.

And finally, to you, the reader. Your curiosity about what we eat and how it's made is what fuels this work.

Thank you for asking questions and for being a curious human being. If you've ever wondered, *"What exactly does a food technologist do?"*, this book is, in part, my answer.

1. Introduction

Why FFS?

For Foods Sake is to remind people that we should be eating real food, not pretend food.

Yes, the title is a play on the acronym "for fucks sake" and this is intentional, because the food industry today really makes me throw my hands up! Why is it that despite advances in technology and innovation in food, each year we seem to be getting sicker and sicker? Why is obesity a huge problem in the developed world? Why are we stuck in a constant struggle with dieting and disease?

Throughout my career as a food technologist, I realised that it doesn't matter how many different types of products we make as an industry, we are still having global health problems, the three diseases of heart disease, obesity and diabetes that plague society, as well as cancer.

Here is the story of why I'm really writing this book.

Before working in the food industry, I absolutely LOVED fried chicken.

When I was 8 years old, I used to eat chicken nuggets all the time. It was my absolute favourite meal at any restaurant.

1. Introduction

So, when I got a job working for one of the biggest poultry suppliers in the nation, it was like a dream come true. As part of my job, I had to sample chicken nuggets, tenders, and wings for quality checks. Every single day. One of my favourite memories was going to fried chicken festivals (yes, this is a thing) where I would go and buy every single fried chicken item from each food truck and assess them on the spot. It meant laying them all out on a table, taking pictures of it, making assessments for its crunchiness, flavour profile, the type of batter it used and also to take any outstanding samples back to the lab.

At first, it was great. But then it wasn't. For some this really is a dream job. Here's the thing, it becomes your job and all that chicken eating is no longer for pleasure. It was my job to ensure that every crunch, every ounce of chicken-y goodness is experienced in every bite of a chicken nugget or tender.

Within weeks, I became depressed and exhausted, and I gained a lot of weight. I gained 5 kilos in just 2 months, my clothes stopped fitting properly, and my chest started to feel tight.

When I saw my doctor, he sat me down and looked me in the eye.

He said if you keep doing what you're doing, you will die.

With a family history of heart disease, this terrified me. I didn't want to end up like my parents, relying on medication to survive.

For Foods Sake

I was only 30 years old at the time.

I did not want to die from CHICKEN NUGGETS!

It dawned on me.

Why was I creating products that were making me, and potentially others sick? Despite my education and expertise, I found myself caught in the very trap I was helping to set.

I started tracing back the steps of how these products were made and marketed.

The more I uncovered, the more I felt I was complicit in something that was very deceptive.

If people knew what I knew, they might start making different choices, choices that could change their lives.

It was also when I started making lifestyle changes that the inspiration for the book came to me.

6 months later, I went back to the doctor for a check-up and he told me, "You might just live a little bit longer".

I wrote this book because I wish it had existed and I had read it before I consumed so many ultra processed foods. I wish it had existed so I could understand what was really going on in the food industry with how foods are made.

1. Introduction

After ten years of working as a food technologist, I realised that for too long, we the consumers have forgotten how to appreciate food. We have lost touch with how our food is made, making it harder to make better decisions for ourselves and our families.

As a food technologist (FT), I loved being able to get the know-how and have an insider's insight into food, food science and the food industry. It's almost like a little secret that FT's have to keep, we know the ingredients, products and processes inside out.

However, being a FT doesn't mean that I'm not a consumer and therein lay the conundrum. As a slightly more aware consumer, I turn a blind eye to certain foods because I enjoy them while some foods I will not eat because I know what goes into them. In a way this has helped me become healthier and more aware of what I put into my body.

As a FT, we work with marketers and salespeople to try to create or 'innovate' where every season there's always a new flavour, variant of something or a brand spanking new product for consumers/customers to spend their money on. Whether it is a health claim or different packaging, the "innovation" doesn't stop.

The more I worked, the more I saw that it didn't matter how many times we 'innovate', every year I see that these diet-related diseases keep rising and creeping up on the global population and the trend is that they don't seem to be going anywhere. It doesn't matter whether a new food product is sugar free, gluten free, paleo, fat free, or full of protein, people are still getting sick and riddled with disease.

Why?

It's because consumers are still ignorant of how to eat or don't know what they put into their mouths and the industry is more than happy to keep them that way. However, this is slowly changing, and the consumers are becoming more aware and knowledgeable.

To be clear, this book isn't a bashing of the food industry, which has seen numerous advances in science and innovation that have benefitted lots of people in the last few decades. However, what's happening is that some companies are more focused on profit than the wellbeing of their customers, and this is where I feel that there is a disconnect.

If this disconnect isn't closed soon, I feel that there will be a greater disparity in the wellbeing of people who consume food and for future generations that are getting increasingly sicker, fatter and dying sooner.

So, what is the solution?

I wondered, what if people knew what I knew, about the industry, how a product is made, and what goes into it, would they change their eating habits?

I believe that with a better understanding and better education of what food is, what calories are and getting to see 'under the hood' of how it all works from someone who has worked in the food industry, things will improve. This book is the first step in making this understanding more available.

This book aims to educate and inform about processed and ultraprocessed foods, how a typical food production business operates, aims to bridge the gap between consumer and manufacturer, and to empower you as a consumer to make better choices at the supermarket.

What is a Food Technologist?

You might be thinking, what even is a food technologist?

I'm a former food technologist with over 10 years in the industry based in Australia and New Zealand. I'll be giving an insider view of what goes on behind the curtain making processed foods. Many books and podcasts have extensive coverage of processed foods however there is nothing from a food industry perspective which provides an objective view of how processed foods are made.

So, I'm writing this book because I want consumers to be more aware of how processed foods are made, how the industry runs, what to look out for and I hope to give consumers an insight that you can't just search for on the internet.

Not many people know what a food technologist is. It's one of those careers and titles that need constant explaining whenever you meet someone new.

The most common question I get asked is "Are you a chef?" or people will simply assume that you must be able to cook well.

Instead, I just say "A food technologist is basically the oompa loompa of any processed food that you see sold in the supermarket. I'm responsible for the taste, packaging, flavours, textures, nutritional panels etc"

The typical response is, "Wow, that's such a cool job!" or "I didn't realise that's a job but now that I think about it, of course it is!" or "That's my dream job!".

When I tell them that I no longer work as a food technologist, people often ask, "Why did you leave? It sounds like an awesome job!".

It was and no doubt there were great aspects to being a food technologist that other jobs simply don't have. Some of these include being paid to eat, going to a food market and buying everything for market research, and trying new flavours of products before they reach the market.

To clarify, I do not represent any companies or organisations. However, this book does draw upon my own experience, other food technologists who have and still work in the industry and peer-reviewed research.

Now that I no longer work in the food industry, I have the freedom to write about an industry which I'm not dependent on drawing a salary or

1. Introduction

career from. Also throw in some millennial burnout and wanting a change in lifestyle, and you'll get the reasons why I left the industry and why I'm no longer a food technologist.

In the process of writing this book, I met with various professionals from doctors, therapists to food addiction coaches who told me that they had clients, who are suffering from eating too much processed or ultra processed foods. They encouraged me to continue writing this book. In a way, I feel that I may have been indirectly contributing to this equation of consumers not being able to make better decisions which led to them making poorer life choices. This doesn't align with my values of wanting to see a healthier world and consumers not being duped by clever marketing. With writing this book, this is my own attempt at redemption for that contribution.

Please do not let me or this book prevent anyone from wanting to join the food industry, it can be rewarding in its own ways especially if you love food and if you're reading this book, I hope this helps you make the decision to join the industry to make a difference.

This book is a synthesis of how the food industry works and how processed food is made.

My experience working in the food industry

My first foray in the food industry really started when I was a child, I honestly just loved all junk and processed foods. I still do to be honest; I love a chocolate chip cookie and a bag of potato crisps. It was my love of food that made me want to become either a chef or baker. However, I realised that being a chef or baker meant anti-social hours, and I was told to study food technology at Massey University in New Zealand by my father and a career adviser.

My bachelor's degree of food technology taught me the nuances of how processed food is made from a scientific and technical perspective. After graduating I worked for both large corporations and small food startups and I learnt a lot from those companies in industries ranging from pet food, poultry, dairy, supplements and chocolate.

I specialised predominantly in new product development, which meant I was the person responsible for creating new types of flavours for products, new range of products (think a new type of Greek style yoghurt). It is very satisfying to see a product that you created on the shelves of a supermarket even after you have left the job. Also, you have great bragging rights to friends as you can point out advertising and billboards and tell them, "I made that". Those were the fun parts of working in the food industry.

1. Introduction

Even in university, I knew that I just wanted to make products and not do anything engineering related (I hated physics). Being able to walk into a supermarket and say "Hey, I made that" is honestly a very cool flex that not many people are able to do. Being able to see how an idea or concept becomes a fully-fledged commercial reality which you can use almost all five senses to really experience is one of the reasons why I became a food technologist in the first place. Even though you're not getting the reputation or credit for the products that you create, you are part of the chain that inadvertently gives energy, drives momentum and creates memories in your community, the industry and in the food products that you create.

Working in various teams means that communication is super crucial. As with any career, it is more important when you are a product developer where there are strict deadlines and launch dates that cannot be missed.

The best thing about being a product developer is being able to taste things that the public will never be able to consume. We are essentially the gatekeepers that ensure that what you have been consuming is of a suitable standard and there is a whole science and industry behind this called sensory science which will be covered later in this book.

Being able to get an inside look into how food products are made is enlightening and fascinating since there are many products, flavours and textures that we simply do not ever get to see as members of the public.

However, the downside of working in the food industry as a product developer meant that you were responsible for the nurturing of your project or the 'baby' and to give it birth and life to the world. This meant doing kitchen and factory trials. The reality of doing factory trials is a necessary evil for any product developer, you must be on site regardless of the time. There have been many times where the factory will call you up at some ungodly hour only for you to arrive at the factory and be told the conveyor belt needs engineering fixing and it will be delayed by another 4 hours.

When factory trials happen, you need to be responsible for every aspect that is happening in the factory. From the temperatures of the vat tanks, the speed of the conveyor belts, how the ingredients are mixed, the storage of the ingredients, how the product is going to be packaged, and the list goes on and on. Even with help from the production/factory staff and depending on the type of product you're working with, this can go smoothly or very wrong.

It is a common joke in the food industry when running factory trials where it is the mother of Murphy's law that if anything can go wrong, it will go wrong. Some of these things can include the machinery breaking down, power cuts, lack of staff, wrong ingredients supplied and sometimes everything all at once.

At a high level, the not so fun parts of being a food product developer was that it is an endless cycle of having to feed the marketing loop and supermarkets' demands for new flavours and "innovation". Regardless of what category of food you're in, there will always be some kind of 'new' flavour or a packaging change that the customer or market wants so as a product developer, you must solve those problems and make sure that your internal and external stakeholders are happy.

This all for the sake that you as a consumer get some delicious product that you simply grab from the supermarket aisles at your convenience.

What does a food technologist do?

The role of a food technologist or a food scientist can range from the following:

New Product Development (NPD)

The innovation of how new foods are made usually comes from the food technologist working alongside the marketing team. NPD must work out the nuances of how a new product can be made in the factory, sourcing the raw materials, conducting trials, ensuring that the product has the right shelf life, sensory properties (taste, texture), nutritional information and ensuring it is cost effective. The NPD career path can be fun as it means you're creating products not yet seen in the supermarket and it often means you're trialling new different types of flavours, texture and packaging that consumers will never get to see.

Quality Assurance

The food industry could not survive without quality assurance. Quality assurance is a set of activities that ensure that quality during the process at which a food is made is met. These activities could include process checklists, project audits etc. These activities are often developed before a product has been made and is not specific to a type of product. Quality assurance is a proactive activity in the food industry and aims to prevent defects of the product before it reaches the consumer.

Quality Control

Quality control is different from quality assurance where it is referring to identifying and rectifying any issues with the product. It is a reactive type of activity as opposed to Quality assurance which is more proactive. Such activities for quality control can include corrective actions to ensure that product defects do not happen again and often liaise with quality assurance to ensure that it is implemented in the process (In most companies, not all of them). For example, a customer calls up and says there's black speck on their bread, which could be a burnt crumb.

Quality control must investigate where that black speck came from and rectify that issue and work with quality assurance to make sure that it doesn't happen again.

In some companies, especially small and medium enterprises (SME), the Quality Control and Assurance responsibilities are rolled into one and are usually split when the workload is too much for one person and/or when the company expands its operations. Quality control and assurance usually have strong skills in statistics to validate if something will go wrong or to prevent a defect from occurring again.

During my time working as a product development technologist, one of the responsibilities was to also conduct quality control of existing products. When you're working in the food industry, it is very easy to put on unnecessary weight. In one of my jobs working in a dairy company, I had to eat the factory's previous batches of yoghurt, flavoured milk, cheese and fresh milk. This meant giving each a pass or fail. If a product didn't taste or feel right, we had to liaise with the quality control/assurance team that something wasn't right.

This often launches an investigation, comparison of other batches and sometimes a complete hold of a production batch before it can be sold to any customers. This is an important step of food production. Ensuring that products have consistent textures, flavours etc takes a team. Sometimes the number of samples that are consumed contains more calories than you need. Hence why there is a spit bucket, where you get to taste the samples without having to ingest them. The spit bucket is an optional tool used in the food industry for those who are health conscious.

Process Technologist

A process technologist is different from a NPD technologist where they focus more on how a food product is made. Process technologists often have engineering backgrounds or the capability to understand how a product can be made in a full-scale production. Process technologists work alongside NPD and Quality to ensure that the equipment, standards and safety measures are met when making the product. Process technologists know the parameters of their equipment such as heat, moisture, run time etc to meet the product specifications.

Packaging Technologist

A packaging technologist is responsible for the design, development and testing of food packaging and to ensure that the food inside the packaging is safe from contamination, can be processed in the factory, and is cost effective. The packaging technologist often works alongside marketing, logistics, quality and production to ensure any new or existing packaging materials are functioning and are fit for purpose.

The entire process of making a food product

Every processed and ultra processed food product is made in a factory or manufacturing plant that has a team of experts in making the food that we all eat. The process of creating a product from ideation to commercialisation is pretty much the same regardless of the food category. The only real nuances are the specific processing, product parameters that are unique to each category such as cheese, beer, yoghurt, muesli bars etc.

1. Introduction

The principles of making a food product are simple yet it can be complex depending on the type of food or beverage that you're wanting to create (Floros et al., 2010). Behind the scenes, food technologists, packaging specialists, quality assurance teams, and engineers work meticulously to ensure the product is safe, consistent, and appealing to consumers. While small businesses sometimes lack resources, they often drive innovation, whereas large corporations are in the business of refining existing products, maintaining the status quo and may occasionally adapt trends to maintain market dominance (Bigliardi & Galati, 2013).

Who is involved

In a large company you would have specific resources or people who would do these roles, for smaller companies, typically a founder or director of a food company would have multiple roles. Each of these roles, while very different, are the 'people' ingredients that make processed food possible.

Technical roles could be product technologists, packaging technologists, quality checks and quality assurance.

Marketing

Love or hate them, marketing is a necessity in the food industry and in business in general. Marketing can be game changing for a food product and is often the deciding factor if a product is successful or not.

Sometimes good food marketing can identify a gap in the market and suggest a flavour that they see from trends and recommend that the technical team make them.

In the food industry, the marketing and product development teams usually work together in tandem. The successful ones can do this seamlessly where they are communicating with each other and have planned product launches in the pipeline.

Sales

This is a role that ensures that your product is seen on the supermarket aisle. Sales or business development roles are important in any business and especially so in a food business. They often can liaise and see what is happening in the supermarket and have the relationships in the industries to ensure they are able to continue seeing products on the supermarket shelves. These roles range from but are not limited to sales reps, business development or category managers.

Procurement

The ingredients must come from another supplier, and the procurement role ensures that the ingredients that are purchased are of the quality and price that the product requires. Procurement plays an important role in ensuring there is a good price negotiated for the ingredients and often works together with the product development team to find the right supplier, ensuring they have the right certifications and paperwork.

Logistics

How your product is stored and arrives at your products distribution centres or warehouses is crucial. While not directly involved in the making of food products, they are an important part of making

1. Introduction

processed food possible. Sometimes packaging technologists will work with logistics to conduct transport trials to ensure they can last the journey to specific locations or conditions.

Finance

Like with every business, you must know your costs of goods, and this is especially true for food products where it is a volume game. Understanding how much your ingredients, packaging, processing, labour costs is part of being in the food business. Typically, the margins in the food business are very small (anywhere between 5-20% and if you're doing more than this in a food business then you're doing great).

Quality

Every successful food business has some form of quality assurance and control; it is a necessity not just to ensure the taste but also food safety. Some food businesses skip on this because they sometimes rely on production to do this but that is not always easy as they require additional training, and it means more workload for production staff.

Production

No food product can be made without production roles, and it is simply the nature of the industry. It is a mixture of equipment and labour that ensures that product is being made. This is usually manual labour that is either directly or indirectly involved in making the food product when it is being scaled up for production. They usually don't have any creative input into the product as the final product recipe from the product development team is given to the production team to create.

Engineering

Because processed food requires some form of automation, machinery or mechanical equipment to create food products at scale, they will break down and require maintenance. In bigger companies, there are dedicated teams who look after the machinery whilst smaller companies would either contract out their engineering departments or have their product teams trained up to have some understanding of the machine and other working parts.

Customer service

Food product inquiries or complaints will inevitably happen, and you will need a customer service representative to be able to explain and answer questions your consumers may have.

The differences between small businesses and big companies

Aside from the obvious accessibility to resources and networks, big corporations typically would have made numerous iterations of their product and taken inspiration from smaller companies and trends so they can keep up and innovate.

The different types of product development

In the food industry, creating food products is a team sport. You need everyone listed above to be onboard and essentially 'buy' into the concept of the new food product that is going to be created.

Typically, this is usually initiated by marketing teams where they should have done their research on the types of products that would be beneficial to the business/company, generate a new market, claw market share from their competition, identify and jump on trends. Not all marketing teams are created equal, and some do more thorough research than others.

For example: When I used to work for a company that made extruded snacks, instead of doing any kind of market research, the marketing team only got perspective and approvals from a certain individual which meant that their marketing efforts for a new product were based on one person's preference as opposed to any grounded research. This product didn't survive 3 months on supermarket shelves.

Product development teams can also come up with different ideas and flavours and suggest it as a potential product.

Product development is both a noun and a verb in the food industry. You have a product development team which does product development.

Stage gate

Product development is usually done as work projects and are managed as such. One such way of managing these projects is the Stage gate process.

The Stage-Gate management process or the Phase-Gate process is a project management technique used to guide a project from conception to launch (Cooper, 2019). It is particularly useful in the development of new food products, such as the different types of product development listed earlier.

The process is divided into stages (or phases), separated by gates. Each stage consists of a set of parallel activities, and each gate serves as a decision point where the project is reviewed and a decision is made to continue, revise, or halt the project to minimise wasted resources. At each gate, especially if it is at a larger corporation or company, would be monitored by a panel that is not directly contributing to that project.

If it's a smaller company, then the gate's decision would typically be determined by the owner or leadership team.

Whenever you see any processed food in the supermarket, as a consumer you will never get to see the many iterations or the revisions of it, packaging trials and sensory tests before it reaches the shelves.

When working as a product development technologist, there was a limited-edition lemon cake

1. Introduction

flavoured milk, and I had to ensure that the flavour was on point and memorable. The company I had worked for had very strict guidelines on what they would allow to be launched, and that is fair enough as you want consumers to have a good experience and come back for more. There were many sensory evaluations trials (explained in a later chapter) to get the one flavour. In the end, there were at least 50 variations of the one flavour before it got released. Some had more lemon, some had more cake taste, it is a process to get a balanced flavour profile that will appeal to the masses.

Branded products (e.g., Coca-Cola) invest heavily in marketing, while private label (supermarket brands) often replicate successful products at lower costs (Hobbs & Young, 2022). Private label products often go through the same process however it will be the supermarket that will give the directive on how the food product will look however the product will be the same, in terms of ingredients. For a private label product to compete with a branded product, they will save costs by reducing distribution and marketing expenses and sometimes using cheaper ingredient substitutes but not always. Think of a private label food product as a strategic replica of successful brand products made by third party suppliers or manufacturers so they can get more market share. Typically, private label food products don't differ majorly from their branded counterparts except for specific flavours, mouthfeel and/or textures.

Become a FOOD DETECTIVE

One of the aims of this book is to help you become a food detective.

What is a food detective? That is what you the reader will become at the end by the time you finish reading this book. A food detective is a consumer that is able to dissect a food product, not be fooled by marketing tricks and able to see a food product with an objective lens to make better health decisions for themselves and their families.

At the end of each specific section of this book, there will be a box of takeaways and snippets of what you should look out for. It will look like this:

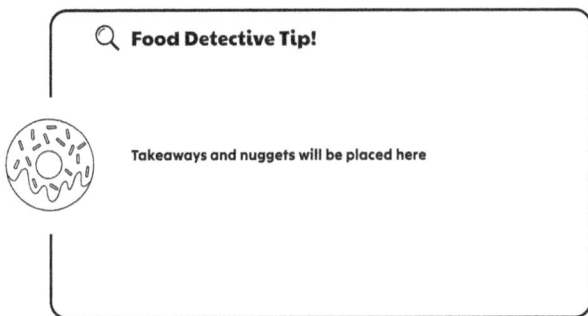

🔍 **Food Detective Tip!**

Takeaways and nuggets will be placed here

2. The definition of food, processed food and ultra processed food

Food is a very broad word, but it is any substance that provides nutrients to the body. Every single animal and living being requires food to sustain itself. This can come from either plant or animal origin and has plenty of tastes, textures, forms in its natural state. Food comes in so many different forms, taste, texture, flavours that the possibilities are boundless. Which is what makes it so magical and creatively infinite.

Food is something that we think about every single day whether you love it or simply loathe the fact that you need to be eating consistently.

Food is great for the simple reason that it allows us to live. Not only that, but it is also a catalyst for bringing people together through bonding and connecting with our history.

The definition of processed food

Over time, food got complicated because we changed it, made it different to suit our ever-changing needs and demands. The definition of a processed food is when food has been altered from its natural state for the purpose of either convenience, safety, and hygiene reasons and/or for easier storage. Processed foods have been around for a long time, and the processing of foods have helped win wars, for example, canned foods and salting meats helped armies survive winter nights.

Even in the food industry, there is no consensus of what processed food is. This book establishes its own definition which you can choose to follow or incorporate into your own current understanding.

What does "processed" mean?

The dictionary meaning of the word processed means to 'to treat or prepare by a particular series of actions'.

One may argue that washing broccoli is processed food but that's just being overtly pedantic. Or is it?

For better or worse, processed food is probably one of the reasons why humans could have survived for so long. If you look at social media posts about processed food, it is getting a bad rep. You're going to get cancer, some disease, you'll become fat and every single detrimental disease that comes with being human. There may be some truth to it but it's best to be objective about what is seen on social media, a lot of those posts have an agenda. It's scare mongering and the food industry does nothing about it because the makers of processed food will probably get shunned for voicing a whisper of an opinion. The exception is clever marketing which this book will delve into, people fall for that all the time.

Without processed food, humanity wouldn't have survived as long as it has. Human history has been driven by ensuring that food is secure, plentiful and able to feed populations. Processed foods mean we're able to withstand droughts, wars, floods etc and because we live in a time where food is no longer scarce, its new forms are so readily available that it has caused unintentional health effects due to its overconsumption.

Of course, that's not what people think when they hear 'processed food', they think about the E-numbers (the e-number, is short for Europe numbers are a codes for permitted substances used in Europe however other countries would just use the numbers without the 'E'), refined grains and glucose syrup used to make it so tasty.

The fact is, we live in a world where processed food is easily available, but at the expense of our wallets and health. In some countries we eat a lot of processed and ultra processed food, and we'll delve into why and whether it still has a place in our lives.

Processed food means that it has been turned into a food product with various processing techniques and where the original food matrix is either maintained, preserved, transformed or manipulated to be either convenient, tasty and or affordable.

What is the food matrix?

The food matrix is the complex physical and chemical structure of food and how its nutrients like protein, fat, carbohydrates are organised and interact with the food's natural given architecture. This architecture and structure are important as it plays a role in how our bodies can digest, absorb and utilise those nutrients.

For example, almond butter and whole almonds almost have almost the same number of macronutrients however the grinding that occurs to make almond butter means that the fats are more readily available to be absorbed whilst the whole almonds have skin and cell walls that the body needs to break down which slows fat absorption. Similarly whole fruit versus juices is an example of where juicing has changed the food matrix because a whole apple's fibre matrix slows sugar absorption, while juicing removes this barrier, leading to a faster blood sugar spike.

One of the reasons why processed foods have its effects on the body is because the food matrix has been altered. It can make nutrients, vitamins and minerals destroyed or more available. Refining wheat into white flour strips away the bran and germ, reducing fibre and mineral absorption, which is why foods like biscuits, muffins etc don't have much fibre content. Foods with an intact matrix (e.g., steel-cut oats) cause slower glucose absorption than their processed counterparts (e.g., instant oatmeal). Fermented foods like yoghurt and kimchi have a modified matrix where microbes predigest some components, enhancing probiotic benefits (Marco et al., 2017).

2. The definition of food, processed food and ultra processed food

The food matrix matters as well to how it satisfies appetite or satiety and how we process the foods in our gastric systems. Foods requiring more chewing (e.g., whole vegetables) increase satiety signals. In contrast, ultra-processed foods (e.g., chips, soft bread) are so easy to eat quickly that they bypass these natural fullness cues (Forde et al., 2013). The body expends more energy digesting whole foods because it must break down the food matrix whilst food processing breaks it down. For example, raw potatoes resist digestion, while cooking gelatinises starch, making it easier to absorb (and higher in available calories). Studies have shown that processed food and ultra processed foods often have *pre-digested* matrices (e.g., hydrolysed proteins, refined flours), requiring less metabolic effort to break down. This may contribute to overeating (Monteiro et al., 2019). So, it is no surprise that diets rich in minimally processed foods (with intact matrices) lower obesity rates, partly because they promote natural portion control (Hall et al., 2019).

How food processing alters the food matrix while sometimes it preserves it

There is an assumption that any processed food must have some kind of additive or 'nasty' to make it the way it is.

This is not always true.

The raw ingredients used for any processed food are very much the same that you would buy from a farmer, supermarket or supplier. The main difference is the ability to scale in a factory and production line as opposed to what you could make at a home kitchen.

Take making blueberry jam as an example.

You're still using ingredients such as blueberries and sugar with the option of adding lemon juice, cinnamon or pectin.

These are all ingredients that you can purchase from a supermarket easily. Even pectin which is actually a naturally occurring thickener that can be found in citrus.

Making jams mostly preserves the food matrix of the blueberries and the difference is companies would have conducted shelf-life trials to ensure it can last up to the best before date and how long it can last when it has been opened.

But if we take another example of something that goes through further processing, like hazelnut spread which is an UPF. These contain ingredients that have significantly changed the food matrix from its original state. Typically, these contain hazelnuts, palm oil, sugars, cocoa powder, an emulsifier and milk powder. All these ingredients again can be obtained from your shops, but you won't be able to replicate what you get store bought because food companies have access to processing and machinery that you cannot simply buy over the shelf.

2. The definition of food, processed food and ultra processed food

The processing of processed food is the intellectual property of that food company and unless it is shown to the public (it usually never is, if it is, it is very brief and general).

Each food company has its own processing measures, parameters, engineering and knowhow that is what makes it different from its competitors. Think of each food manufacturer as a 'chef'. If you give different chefs the same ingredients and ask them to create the same dish, it will inevitably be different. If you go to a café and order an eggs benedict and a coffee, it will come out differently. The eggs benedict may have a different hollandaise sauce, no one knows how that hollandaise sauce is made, only the chef knows, and this is the same for food manufacturers.

The main difference with food manufacturing is that there are strict laws, regulations and quality checks before it can even reach the supermarket.

With the hazelnut spread example, you can make it at home however how you grind the hazelnut, the order in which you put the ingredients, how you blend those ingredients together, the temperature at which you add them in, the type of sugar you add, will make a difference to the taste, cost and quality of that product.

There is food processing that helps preserve the food matrix in the form of freezing, roasting or washing where the nutrient loss is minimal and usually the fibre and cellular structures remain largely intact.

So, the next time you see the same types of products on the supermarket shelf, look at the manufacturer and think about how it could be made.

The 'chefs' in food manufacturing isn't just one person, it's often a group of people and teams to make that product tasty, affordable and packaged for your convenience.

Ultra processed food (UPF) and processed food are essentially food ingredients that have been pre-digested for you, and the body doesn't have to do as much work or use as much energy to break it down. However, these ingredients need ingredients to supplement them to ensure they are palatable. That's where added sugars, fats and salts come in.

The food matrix also explains why a "calorie is not just a calorie", where two seemingly similar foods with almost the same nutrient profiles will have very different effects on your body because of how it is processed. This is why there is a recommendation of eating more whole foods, which really means eat more foods that have their food matrix intact.

Why do processed foods exist?

Human beings would not have survived without processing their food and we have done so since the prehistoric ages when humans first began making tools. Whether it be catching a mammoth and cooking it over a fire or salt preservation, food processing is in our DNA.

2. The definition of food, processed food and ultra processed food

The reason why it exists is for several reasons and mainly because they benefit us:

Preservation – Processed foods last longer than fresh foods. Whether it is heat or chemical treatment with the use of salt or preservatives, this kills off any harmful bacteria and microorganisms that otherwise could be present in it.

Distribution – Because processed food lasts longer, it can travel further which makes it possible for everyone to eat things from the other side of the world.

Convenience – Preparing fresh food means that you usually process it yourself which can take a long time where we live in a fast-paced world and not many are able to grow their own garden or cook their own meals and there's not many natural foods that require little preparation (except for bananas and certain nuts but even to a certain degree they have been processed as well).

Cheaper – Sometimes because certain foods have been processed in large volumes, this can often make them more affordable for the end consumer and especially profitable for the manufacturer. Because certain foods have been processed, convenience is what consumers pay for.

Availability – Processed foods allow for poorer countries to get nutrition that would otherwise be unavailable to them and helps with food shortages or nutritional deficiencies.

Taste – Fresh food is great but sometimes processed food is transformed to deliver such an extraordinary sensory experience that otherwise can't be replicated in nature (such as chocolate).

Appearance – Processed food can be made to look appealing to us in a way that natural foods can't. When food is processed, it can be presented to be appealing with the use of different ingredients and processing techniques. This also helps food manufacturers differentiate themselves from the competition and a recognisable appearance is good for marketing. If it looks pretty enough, you'll want to try it.

Categories of processed foods

Fresh foods or minimally processed foods	Fresh or frozen fruit and vegetables, raw meat, nuts, seeds
Primary processed or refined foods (1°)	Rice, pasta, sugar
Secondary processed foods (2°)	Butter, flour, oils
Tertiary processed foods (3°)	Canned fruits, vegetables, fish, peanut butter
Ultra processed foods (UPF)	Typically have additives and the food matrix is no longer intact

Fresh Food/Ingredients or minimally processed foods

This is self-explanatory. However, the 'process' involving fresh food and ingredients is minimal and usually only involves cleaning, washing, dehulling of shells/husks or temperature storage. Natural foods that tend to deteriorate faster than most of these foods include:

2. The definition of food, processed food and ultra processed food

- Fresh Fruit

- Vegetables

- Nuts and seeds are a great processed food, they are processed to be able to access the nutrients from its natural state. Cashews for example look very different from the natural state from what you get in the supermarket.

- Raw meat

- Frozen foods such as frozen fruits and vegetables retain the freshness and nutrients of those foods and last longer than fresh fruits and vegetables

Primary Processed/Refined Food (1^0)

These are defined as ingredients or 'staples' that you'd find in most kitchens and pantries and usually involved another form of process or cooking such as grinding, refining, sieving, moulding, or heat treatment:

- Rice

- Pasta

- Sugar

- Salt/Pepper

- Oats are also a great processed food that gives fibre, protein and vitamins that has many health benefits.

Secondary (2⁰) processed food

These are processed food ingredients where typically you aren't going to eat them by themselves. These can include oils, butter, sugar and salt.

These are usually used in combination with other ingredients.

And typically, they have been used by humans for thousands of years just in various forms. Take flour as an example, you wouldn't eat flour by itself, but you need it and other processed culinary ingredients to make ultra processed food.

Tertiary (3⁰) processed food

These are foods that have taken fresh raw materials and processed them to last longer but are still close to their raw form.

- Canned fruits and vegetables

- Canned fish such as salmon and tuna are great alternatives to fresh varieties to those who can't afford it and still retain the nutrients.

- Salted nuts

- Hummus

- Peanut butter

These have been processed for preservation usually by heating, salting or smoking. These foods were made for convenience or for a longer shelf life.

Ultra processed foods

Ultra processed foods or UPF are foods that consist of secondary and sometimes primary and tertiary processed foods with additives to make it more appealing to the sensory experience. Such additives include flavours, emulsifiers, thickeners, sweeteners and oils.

UPF is also the new terminology for "junk food". The term "junk food" first appeared in the 1970s then until roughly the 2010s, when "ultra-processed foods" began replacing it in scientific and policy circles. Whilst the term "junk food" has not been completely superseded, it is still used in everyday language. The term UPF originated from Brazilian nutrition researcher Carlos Monteiro and colleagues began using the concept of food "processing" to explain dietary risks that weren't fully captured by nutrient-based labels. Monteiro introduced the NOVA food classification system, which defined "ultra-processed foods" (UPFs) as industrial formulations with multiple ingredients, additives, and processing steps. This classification system is still being reviewed and the categories described previously are loosely based on that.

UPF typically does not resemble the original food source it is derived from, so the original food matrix has been completely changed. Or it will be processed so much just to mimic the look of the food's natural state, for example, certain crisps that have been shaped to resemble a vegetable.

UPFs often comprise the Irresistible Tri Factor of fat, sugar, and salt.

From my experience working in the food industry, there are different types of ultra processed foods. I'm going to break them down even further:

UPF Primary

These are basically the tertiary category of processed food but could just have a little bit of flavour, seasoning just to give it an extra oomph that is not required but is often added to give it a unique selling point. An example of this is salted peanuts with chilli seasoning which then has additional salt and flavouring to make it more addictive.

UPF Addict

These are foods that are designed to make you addicted to them, think of chips/crisps, cookies. These are usually a combination of fat, sugar, salt (the Irresistible Tri Factor) and a texture that is crunchy or crispy that tells our brain that it is "good" for us. These are specifically designed for maximum sensory experience that our primitive ape brains just can't get enough of.

UPF Decadence

These are foods that are made to give a sense of luxury and decadence, think of chocolate, puddings, ice cream, etc. The main factor of UPF decadence is their mouthfeel, ingredients such as cocoa, vanilla, high fat and sugar content. Not as addictive as the UPF addict foods but something that you would consider as a 'treat'. UPD Decadence foods can also be addictive as well.

UPF Culturally ingrained

Some foods are part of the culture and cuisine, even if it is ultra processed. Some of these include branded malt chocolate powder, breads, muffins, certain biscuits or cookies.

UPF Added benefit/Supplements/Protein bars etc

Supplements, protein bars, gels are foods that are technically ultra processed but because they have an added benefit of extra protein, BCAAs (Branched chain amino acids), creatine or something fitness related they are usually not given the same scrutiny as other UPFs.

UPF convenience

Everything that has been processed into a format and size that makes it portable, easy to open and consume on the go ranging from chocolate, coke, frozen TV dinners and microwave popcorn. The products here have been so processed that there are little natural nutrients left and would have been supplemented with vitamins and or minerals after the fact.

The Cons of Processed Food - Why certain processed foods are detrimental

Processed food comes in different shapes, forms, sizes and categories.

Over time, processed foods were manufactured not for the benefit of keeping consumers fed but because of a focus on profit over people. This led to companies creating processed foods that were lacking nutrients and with maximum sensory experience in taste, flavour and texture. The food industry knows that humans are creatures of habit and used this to their advantage where they created foods that are high in the Irresistible Tri Factor of fat, sugar and salt which meant they had a high chance of returning customers, which results in higher profits. This meant that processed foods were detrimental for the reasons below:

Loss of vitamins and minerals – In some foods, the naturally occurring vitamins and minerals have been completely stripped away once processed. The processing can be done through heating (usually this is the case), physical disintegration (E.g. frying, extruding) of the natural food matrix (this means that the micronutrients can no longer be held together in a state that will make it digestible for humans).

2. The definition of food, processed food and ultra processed food

Use of unnecessary food additives – This is a Catch-22 where additives can help make food taste better, last longer or change its texture however these additives can have detrimental effects to certain individuals. Now the use of food additives is NOT detrimental in the sense that they are going to actively harm you. The quantities used in food additives are minute and so tiny that it is almost impossible to prove if they are having a detrimental effect on you in the long term. Some processed foods have more additives than is required and are added for the sake of increasing profit margins such as thickeners in certain foods like ice cream, yoghurt etc.

High fat, sugar or salt (Irresistible Tri Factor) content – The fat, sugar and salt content in certain processed foods especially fast food often exceeds our recommended daily intake for that nutrient by multiples. Your body simply doesn't need that much all in one go and your brain will be conditioned to believe that the amounts you are eating are perfectly fine. UPF typically has high quantities of one or a combination of these.

Our ancestors previously had to hunt, gather, forage and kill to get their calories from sources like animals, beehives, berries which also meant that we were expending calories to get them (in essence, we had to work for our food). Now with technology in our hands, we can order our meals and groceries from our sofa.

Refined – many processed foods are basically **pre-digested** thus making it easier for your body to absorb which can mean that the body gets the nutrients straight away. However, it also means that the body does not need to work as hard to digest certain foods.

So how are manufactured processed foods created? The following chapters will outline how they are made, how a food business operates, and you can apply the same principles if you're looking to reduce your consumption of UPF.

3. The FFS Framework

The best things come in 3s - So now it's time to introduce the Three Tri Factors of FFS (For Foods Sake)!

Obviously, FFS is a play on the colloquial saying "for fucks sake", while it is a saying that invokes either what we feel should be obvious, something isn't done in a way we want it to, something has caused disappointment or all the above. For me, it is a reminder that food is more than just something to put in our mouths, it is meant to provide meaningful nutrition both mentally and physically. The mental nourishment I hope will come from the learnings in this book.

One of the main objectives of this book and my mission is to get consumers more aware of what happens in the food industry.

One of the ways I have done this is by using a framework called the Tri Factors. The tri factors is a series of frameworks that touch on the different aspects of how processed food is made. The reason they are called tri factors is because there are typically 3 factors that consumers need to look at when they're purchasing processed food, starting from the product itself (what makes it irresistible), the external (marketing), and internally as a consumer (what drives your consumption of processed food). These have been distilled from a mixture of my own experience being a consumer, a product developer and from peer reviewed literature.

In this book, there are 3 main tri factors that will be explored which are:

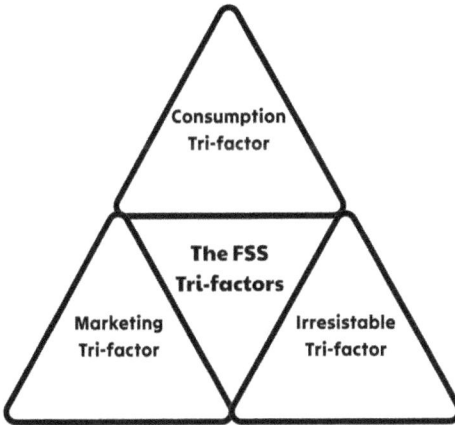

Irresistible Tri Factor

The Irresistible Tri Factor consists of fat, sugar and salt and it explores how this combination has been used for many years to create our greatest and most addictive food products, why they are such a great combination, how to recognise that we're eating too much of it and why it has caused so much strife in the world, and what the food industry is doing to reduce it. We will look at these nutrients separately and how they do play a role in our bodies but also what happens when we consume too much of them.

Marketing Tri Factor

The Marketing Tri Factor is about how consumers are roped into buying processed and ultra processed foods. This will delve into the way marketing has manipulated consumers by using psychology to make products seem either 'healthier' or 'cleaner' when they're not. This causes consumers to buy products that they don't really need and just fill their stomach with empty calories. The Marketing Tri Factor will look into how claims work on the front of the pack, the language of food marketing and to give you an objective lens to not be fooled by food marketing.

Consumption Tri Factor

The Consumption Tri Factor looks deep into the factors of why we consume and purchase the foods that we do. Looking at the taste, price and convenience of a food is what we do subconsciously. Now, armed with new information, I will help break down how you can get the best value for your buck and whether you can gauge if the convenience you're paying for a certain food is worth it. The Consumption Tri Factor will also look into how to factor in your lifestyle when purchasing processed foods based on price, your taste preferences and convenience.

4. The Irresistible Tri Factor

This chapter delves into the compounds in processed and ultra processed food that makes them so irresistible!

Notice that it's very hard to jut eat just one crisp or chip?

The food industry is very aware that for products to be profitable, the more palatable and closer to irresistible, they know that it is worth manufacturing and that they have a business.

The main components that make up the Irresistible Tri Factor are Fat, Sugar and Salt.

Almost all ultra processed food has at least one of these three components in some sort of form or as an ingredient.

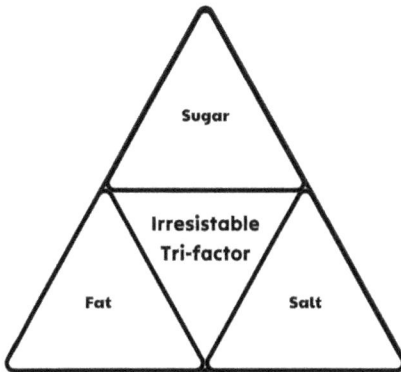

Fat, Sugar and Salt

The Irresistible Tri Factor of fat, sugar, and salt is also the same irresistible trio that is used in restaurants, cafes and Quick Service Restaurants (QSRs). This combination is called the Irresistible Tri Factor because when put together alongside certain mouthfeels and textures of food products, the food products become simply hard to resist. The food industry uses this to their advantage so you, the consumer, have no choice but to succumb to it because of your physiology.

The food that we consider to be delicious, 'bomb', tasty, yummy and all the adjectives all have some tri factor in them that makes them so good to eat. And sometimes each of the tri factors individually are more than enough to make the processed food taste great.

I will also go over the essential factor that is carbohydrates in a later chapter.

Now let's go over each of the Irresistible Tri Factors:

Fat, the carrier of flavour

Fat is a macronutrient required to keep skin healthy, store energy, support hormone function and without it, we cannot live.

However, we have an easy access to fat (our love of anything crispy, creamy, or deep-fried) and with a high prevalence of obesity in developed and developing countries, we are probably eating more fat than we need.

Here is a breakdown of the different types of fat:

Saturated Fat

Think of coconut oil and bacon grease. These are fats that become solid at room temperature. Whilst okay in moderate amounts, they do increase your risk of heart disease. These fats have been demonised for decades, mainly because excessive intake raises LDL (aka "bad") cholesterol, which is linked to heart disease. The issue? Saturated fats are usually in the yummy treat foods like ice cream, cookies, bacon, and fries. Basically, if your taste buds cheer, it probably has saturated fat.

There will be another chapter that delves deeper in the specifics of monounsaturated, polyunsaturated and trans-fat.

Fat was the enemy back in the day

Back in the 90s, fat was touted as the 'enemy' in mass media which led to products to be made 'fat free'. Some of these products still exist and have made food manufacturers put in additional sugars and additives to mimic the 'fat' flavour without the fat.

Fats are preferred by animals including ourselves as a macronutrient because it gives us more calories per gram and it gives us mouthfeel and creaminess that can't be achieved with sugar or salt. Despite the bad rep fats have had over the past few decades particularly the early 90s and 2000s, it has now experienced a turnaround of being the macro that is no longer feared but embraced instead.

The issue with the developed and Western world is that a lot of the processed and ultra processed foods have more saturated and trans-fat than we need in our diet at any given time.

Foods high in saturated fat and trans-fat are typically also the tastiest foods.

However, it's not the saturated fats or trans fats but the mono and poly-unsaturated fats that have been given the limelight as being the hero of the fat family, so to speak.

Even in the restaurant industry, fat is used generously to get you hooked on their dishes. This is also used in the manufactured food industry.

Fat is also a great carrier for flavour, when mixed and fused with other flavour particles, it helps amplify it in different dimensions. Think of ice cream, a fatty combination of cream, sugar and milk (if made like it used to be) and when we have vanilla added to it, it's a very different product. To the point that vanilla ice cream is the 'default' ice cream flavour. No one buys 'plain' ice cream, it would taste creamy, like whipped cream.

Fat also has its imposters too which are the margarines, hydrogenated oils, these were all created to make sure that there would be easily available and cheaply made fat sources for the masses. Cream, butter and coconut oil are natural sources of fat, but they are expensive and time consuming to produce. The "imposter fats" were marketed as healthier alternatives, but many of them contained trans fats that we now know were far worse than the saturated fats they replaced (Lichtenstein et al., 1998).

If a company wanted to replace butter, they would use vegetable fat or shortening to make sure it's cheaper and has a similar taste to the full butter version. You will see this in biscuits or cookies where butter is replaced with margarine to replicate that same buttery taste and mouthfeel.

Why was coconut deemed to be 'unhealthy' in the 90s?

In the 1990s, coconut oil was often viewed as unhealthy primarily in Western countries due to its high saturated fat content. At the time, saturated fats were widely believed to contribute to heart disease by raising levels of LDL cholesterol (often referred to as "bad" cholesterol). This belief was based on the prevailing dietary guidelines and research of that era, which emphasised reducing overall fat intake, particularly saturated fats, to lower the risk of cardiovascular disease.

However, many Eastern and Polynesian nations and countries had been using coconut products for cooking and for skincare for many years before it had been adopted by Western countries as something that was seen as 'healthy' and acceptable in the use of other diets such as ketogenic, vegan etc.

Coconut oil contains about 90% saturated fat, which is significantly higher than many other oils and fats. As a result, it was lumped together with other sources of saturated fats, such as butter and lard, and was often discouraged by health professionals and nutritionists.

However, more recent research has helped clarify that not all saturated fats are equal, and the specific types of saturated fats in coconut oil (medium-chain triglycerides or MCTs) may have different metabolic effects compared to long-chain triglycerides found in other saturated fats. Some research indicates that MCTs can raise HDL cholesterol (often referred to as "good" cholesterol) and may have other health benefits, though the overall impact on heart health remains a topic of debate (St-Onge & Jones, 2002).

Many processed and ultra-processed foods are loaded with excess saturated and trans fats, contributing to rising rates of obesity and cardiovascular disease. It's also one of the reasons why saturated fat is shown in all nutritional labelling to make it clear how much there is.

Sugar is seen as the big devil, but this wasn't always the case. What changed?

Sugar has a long and antiquated history, and it wasn't until in recent years that sugar was even considered a commodity. A lot of history and colonisation is tied into the story of sugar because of the sugar plantations, cane sugar in particular.

Origins of sugar

Sugar, primarily in the form of sucrose, is a natural carbohydrate derived from plants, most notably sugarcane and sugar beets. Its history dates back thousands of years. Sugarcane was first domesticated in New Guinea around 8000 BCE and later spread to Southeast Asia and India. By 500 BCE, Indians developed techniques to crystallize sugar, creating granulated sugar (Galloway, 2005). Sugar cultivation spread to the Middle East and Mediterranean regions through trade routes. During the European colonization of the Americas, sugarcane plantations were established in the Caribbean and South America, driven by the transatlantic slave trade.

Today, sugar is extracted from sugarcane or sugar beets through a process of milling, purification, and crystallization.

It is one of the most widely produced and traded commodities globally.

Sugar is used as a cheap and easy way to increase the palatability of a food, and this has been so for many years.

4. The Irresistible Tri Factor

Uses in the food industry

Sugar is a versatile ingredient with numerous applications in the food industry:

Sweetening: It is used to enhance the flavour of foods and beverages, from soft drinks to baked goods.

Preservation: Sugar acts as a preservative in jams, jellies, and canned fruits by reducing water activity and inhibiting microbial growth.

Texture and structure: In baking, sugar contributes to the texture, moisture, and browning of products like cakes and cookies.

Fermentation: Sugar is a key ingredient in the fermentation processes, such as brewing beer and making bread.

Balancing flavours: It counteracts sourness, bitterness and acidity in foods like tomato sauce and salad dressings, creating a more balanced taste.

Why Sugar is so prevalent

Sugar's ubiquity in modern diets can be attributed to several factors:

Historical trade and economics: The colonial sugar trade made sugar widely available and affordable, transforming it from a luxury item to a household staple.

Industrialisation: Advances in food processing and mass production made sugary foods and beverages cheap and accessible.

Marketing and consumer demand: Aggressive marketing by food companies has promoted sugary products, especially to children, creating a cultural preference for sweet flavour profiles.

Addictive qualities: Sugar's effects on the brain which activates pathways attributed with reward has contributed to its widespread consumption (Lenoir et al., 2007).

Why Humans Can't Resist Sugary Foods

Humans are biologically predisposed to crave sugar due to evolutionary and physiological factors which haven't changed that much:

Evolutionary advantage: In prehistoric times, sweet-tasting foods (like ripe fruits) were safe and energy-dense, providing a survival advantage. Our ancestors evolved to seek out and prefer sweet flavours. Not only that, in the ancestral environment, sweet foods were traditionally rare and or required some form of energy to acquire. Think of a bee's nest to access honey, our ancestors didn't just buy honey, they had to grab it from a tree, fend off dangerous bees with no bug spray and still dig out the honey from the hive.

4. The Irresistible Tri Factor

Brain chemistry: Sugar triggers the release of dopamine, a neurotransmitter associated with pleasure and reward. This creates a "feel-good" response, reinforcing the desire for sugary foods (DiFelice Antonio et al., 2012).

Energy source: Sugar is a quick source of glucose, sugar provides immediate energy, which the body prioritises for survival or use during physical or mental exertion or activity.

Addiction-like effects: Overconsumption of sugar can lead to tolerance, where more sugar is needed to achieve the same pleasurable effect, mimicking addictive behaviours and a hallmark of addictive substances (Avena, Rada, & Hoebel, 2008).

The allure of Carbs

We humans don't just crave sugar, we crave carbohydrates, especially the refined and processed kind. Carbohydrates or carbs is a macronutrient (the other two macronutrients being protein and fat) to give you energy to function and it consists of fibre, starches and sugars. **Sugar is a simple form of carbohydrate** whilst fibre and starches are complex carbohydrates.

A simple carbohydrate can be easily digested and absorbed which leads to a quick rise in blood sugar while a complex carbohydrate takes longer for your body to digest and releases energy in a slower and stable manner (Gropper & Smith, 2021).

Almost every culture in the world has developed their own kind of carb that is uniquely theirs (either a mixture of simple or complex carbohydrates). The principle of carbs being a staple in any diet around the world makes sense and here's why:

Carbohydrates as survival fuel: Carbs are the body's preferred energy source. When metabolised, they provide glucose, critical for both muscular and brain function (Ludwig & Ebbeling, 2018).

Refined carbohydrates and reward: Refined carbs (like white flour, syrups, and starches) are digested rapidly, spiking blood glucose and triggering a dopamine response not unlike sugar's effects (Gearhardt et al., 2011).

Fat + Sugar + Salt = Hyper-Palatability: This trio doesn't occur often in nature, but in processed food, it's engineered to be irresistible. These combinations hijack the brain's reward systems, overriding satiety signals and encouraging overeating (Bliss, 2010). Examples like doughnuts, chips or crisps, chocolate bars and ice cream.

Convenience and emotional eating: Processed carbs are quick to prepare, shelf-stable, and provide comfort in times of stress which contribute to emotional dependency, habitual overconsumption and binge eating.

Health implications

While sugar is a natural part of the human diet, excessive consumption is linked to health issues such as obesity, type 2 diabetes, heart disease, and dental cavities. Public health efforts are increasingly focused on reducing sugar intake through education, labelling, and taxes on sugary beverages (World Health Organization, 2015).

Sugar's journey from a rare luxury to a global staple reflects its deep integration into human culture and diet. Its sweet taste, energy-boosting properties, and ability to enhance food make it irresistible, but its overconsumption poses significant health challenges. However, life would not be sweet without a bit of sugar, so long as we understand how it works in our bodies, how it is used in the food industry, we can make some better decisions for our health.

Salt, is western society eating too much of it? Why do we love salt?

Salt is the original additive, ever since its discovery long before there was modern technology, many civilisations used salt to preserve food and enhance flavour.

However, over the years, salt was used just like sugar to get consumers hooked on food products. This led to the palates of Western consumers having higher intakes of salt than the rest of the world where the average intake is 8 to 12 grams per day when the World Health Organisation (WHO) recommends only 5 grams per day. Historically, salt was used as a currency. Now it may cost us our health instead.

Now the food industry is reducing the salt content in its food products, and they have been doing so for many years. Bread products used to have high salt content, and some companies have reduced their salt content by 10% year on year so that the consumers will not notice the difference.

Food companies are aware of public health campaigns urging salt reduction. The tricky bit for the industry and food technologists is if they reduce salt too quickly from products, we as consumers will notice. So, they reduce it gradually, around 10% per year in some cases so that our taste buds can recalibrate (He et al., 2013). This is not an advertised practice at all except for when there is a specific marketing claim to say, 'lower sodium'.

Origins and composition of salt

Salt, primarily composed of sodium chloride (NaCl), is an essential mineral that has played a crucial role in human civilization. It is necessary for bodily functions such as fluid balance, nerve signalling, and muscle contraction.

Humans have harvested salt for thousands of years, using it for both dietary and preservation purposes. It was used in China as early as 6000 BCE, in Egypt for mummification and preservation, and by the Romans for everything from seasoning to paying the army.

Today, salt is obtained through three primary methods:

Evaporation of seawater (sea salt).

Mining from underground deposits (rock salt).

Extraction from salt flats and brine wells (solar salt).

Salt is widely used in food, industry, and chemical production.

Types of salt:

Table Salt

Highly refined and processed with added anti-caking agents. Often fortified with iodine to prevent iodine deficiency disorders.

Sea Salt

Derived from evaporated seawater. Contains trace minerals that can slightly affect taste and colour.

Himalayan Pink Salt

Mined from ancient salt deposits in the Himalayas. Contains small amounts of minerals like iron, giving it a pink hue.

Kosher salt

Large, flaky crystals that dissolve easily. Common in cooking for seasoning and curing meat.

Rock Salt

Coarse, unrefined salt used for de-icing and some culinary applications.

Salt comes in a rainbow of textures and colours, and with a surprising variety of marketing pitches. Some are sold as healthier alternatives due to their trace minerals, but nutritionally speaking, most salts deliver roughly the same amount of sodium.

Uses in the food industry

Salt has a wide range of functions in food production and culinary practices:

Flavour Enhancement: Intensifies and balances flavours in both sweet and savoury dishes.

Preservation: Prevents microbial growth in foods like cured meats, pickles, and cheeses.

Texture Improvement: Strengthens gluten in baking and controls fermentation in bread making.

Brining and Tenderizing: Helps retain moisture in meats and seafood

Do we eat too much salt?

The short answer is yes; we do, especially in Western societies. And no, most of that isn't from sprinkling salt on your dinner. Over 75% of the salt we consume comes from processed and restaurant foods.

Breads, sauces, ready meals, instant noodles, and takeaway pizzas are major culprits. In fact, bread is one of the top contributors to sodium intake, not because it's particularly salty, but because we eat so much of it.

Health Implications

While salt is necessary for survival, excessive intake is associated with health risks:

Hypertension: The leading risk factor for heart disease and stroke (Appel et al., 2011).

Kidney disease: Salt overconsumption strains the kidneys, leading to long-term damage.

Water retention: Consuming too much salt may cause bloating and swelling and could be why the rings on your fingers feel tight after a takeaway feast.

For individuals genetically predisposed to salt sensitivity, even moderate excess can be damaging. That's millions of people walking around with pressure building in their veins sometimes unknowingly.

Salt is an indispensable part of human history, cuisine, and physiology. While moderate salt intake is essential for health, excessive consumption which is largely driven by processed foods has been a health risk for several decades now.

How mouthfeel and texture make us addicted to processed foods

It's not just the Irresistible Tri Factor of fat, sugar and salt that makes us consumers addicted to UPF. There is another powerful layer of irresistibility into processed and ultra-processed foods: specific mouthfeels and textures which some food technologists and scientists have engineered to give us that desirable OOHMF or CRUNCH.

Attributes like crunchiness, creaminess, and meltability are meticulously designed to create a highly pleasurable and memorable sensory experience that keeps consumers coming back for more. Upon saying that, some of these experiences are what make food exciting. However, it does become an issue when it becomes additive.

The Neuroscience of "Mouthfeel"

The appeal of texture is not merely psychological; it is deeply rooted in our human biology.

The sound of crunch is a powerful signal of freshness and quality. Research has shown that our perception of crispness is intensely influenced by the sound a food makes when we bite it. This sonic feedback, often amplified in products like chips, crackers, and crispy cereals, triggers a heightened sensory response. The brain associates this loud, satisfying crunch with a food that is at its peak, making the experience more stimulating and rewarding (Spence, 2015). This is why a stale chip is so profoundly disappointing, it fails to deliver on the expected auditory and textural promise and only gives dissatisfaction.

For food technologists, this is the field of rheology where it is measuring how materials form and deform under pressure. It is like mechanical testing where bending, compression or fracturing play a part in quantifying crunchiness in crisps, biscuits and even apples.

Food scientist Steven Witherly, in his book *Why Humans Like Junk Food*, highlights two key concepts:

Dynamic contrast: This occurs when a food presents two or more contrasting textures simultaneously. A classic example is the chocolate-coated ice cream: a hard, crispy shell giving way to a cold, creamy interior. This contrast makes the eating experience more complex and interesting than a single, uniform texture, compelling the brain to pay more attention and derive more pleasure from the experience. For consumers, time tends to slow down as your brain is taking in this new information and experience.

Vanishing caloric density: Witherly identifies this as a key trait of many addictive foods. These are foods that melt or dissolve quickly in the mouth (e.g., cheese puffs, extruded snacks, ice cream, certain biscuits). The rapid disappearance tricks the brain into thinking it's consuming fewer calories than it really is. The oral sensors tell the brain, "It's gone already, you must not have eaten much," which short-circuits our natural fullness cues and encourages overconsumption (Witherly, 2007).

Smooth, creamy textures, often achieved with emulsifiers, fats, and gums, are inherently comforting. This texture is subconsciously linked to high-fat, energy-dense foods like mother's milk or ripe fruit, which are vital for survival. Some processed foods and UPF exploit this primal preference in products like chocolate spreads, creamy yoghurts, whipped toppings, and melt-in-the-mouth biscuits. The luxurious coating sensation is highly palatable and encourages repeated consumption to re-experience that comfort.

How does this all create a food product "hook"?

The combination of these engineered textures creates a powerful feedback loop:

1. **Sensory-specific satiety:** Humans experience something called "sensory-specific satiety," where we become full and bored of a specific flavour or texture. UPFs are designed to overcome this. By offering complex layers of flavour *and* contrasting textures (e.g., a chewy cookie with crunchy chips and a creamy filling), they continuously stimulate the palate, delaying feelings of boredom and allowing us to eat a larger volume before feeling satiated (Public Health Collaboration, 2022).

2. **The repeatable experience:** Unlike whole foods, where an apple's crunch or a carrot's snap can vary, the texture of a processed food is uniform, consistent and predictable. Every single chip

from a packet delivers almost the exact same crunch. This reliability creates a strong learned preference. The consumer knows exactly what rewarding sensation to expect, building brand loyalty and a repetitive purchasing habit.

3. **The absence of effort:** Whole foods often require significant chewing effort (e.g., a tough cut of meat, raw vegetables). Processed foods are typically engineered for easy eating; they are soft enough to eat quickly but textured enough to be interesting. This low effort/high reward ratio facilitates rapid eating, often before the body's signals of fullness (which take about 20 minutes to register) have had a chance to kick in.

The pursuit of the perfect "crunch," "cream," or "melt" is a deliberate and sophisticated science. By leveraging our innate sensory preferences for freshness, energy density, and variety, food manufacturers create products that are not just tasty but sensorially captivating. This engineered texture, combined with optimised flavours and guilty pleasure marketing, makes UPFs highly difficult to resist, playing a significant role in their addictive potential and contributing to their overconsumption.

How the Irresistible Tri Factor causes so much strife in the world

The FSS (Fat, Sugar and Salt) Irresistible Tri Factor is a sensorial, mathematical, physiological and scientific masterpiece that humans struggle to resist. Whether it's in a restaurant or a factory, this is a winning combination that makes people come back consistently to eat food products. It is also called the 'bliss point', 'hyper-palatability' or what I like to call the 'X factor' where fat, sugar, and salt work so well that food becomes irresistible (Kessler, 2009). Combine this with a mouthfeel or crunchy texture, and this becomes a gateway for continuous consumption.

And it is very profitable for business and for that reason, it is not commonly told to consumers faces that this is happening to them. Yet, the food industry's reliance on these ingredients is no secret.

The FSS combo combined with the textural and mouthfeel experiences make certain foods completely irresistible to most consumers. Think of crisps, cookies and chips. You can't just have one of these, you will keep eating these especially if they are sitting right in front of you on a desk, at a party or when you are binge watching some series or a movie.

The reason why this has caused so much strife in the world is because our primitive monkey brains have not evolved fast enough to discern what is 'food or sustenance' and 'food-like substances' which are very different from one another. Our brains are still wired for environments where calories are scarce and the FSS Irresistible Tri Factor is seen as a rare ultimate prize. Your brain is going to want that ultimate prize every time, it doesn't know you haven't worked for it like our ancestors did. Ultra processed food triggers the same signals of naturally occurring fat, sugar signals energy dense nutrients and salt is needed for essential bodily functions. So, our tastebuds tell our brains to register certain tastes, mouthfeel and sensations as more beneficial.

This makes these food-like substances very addictive, satisfying and can make us forgo our original sources of food such as fruits and vegetables which will seem inferior when it comes to a sensory experience for some consumers.

The FSS combo often strips the food ingredients of their original matrix, vitamins, minerals and when we consume these products, our bodies believe that those micronutrients will be there because of the similar sensory cues. However, oftentimes, we do not know or are not in tune with our bodies to know that we are causing them harm. This causes a disconnect between what our bodies think they need versus what they are actually getting nutritionally. Over time this disconnect is widening further as natural whole foods start to pale in comparison to the eating experience of ultra processed foods. Strawberries' sweetness pales in comparison to a lollipop or a chocolate bar and a handful of almonds pales in comparison to the hot, crunchy, salty goodness of French fries. This makes our preferences sway towards ultra processed foods over whole foods instead.

Whenever you can, opt for whole foods first that still have the food matrix intact over food-like substances that are giving you a sensory dopamine hit.

What are additives and are they that scary?

Food additives or what are sometimes called "nasties" by various food marketing campaigns and influencers are an important part of food in general and not just processed food.

Food additives have a function first and foremost to ensure that the food we consume is safe or meets the needs of the consumer whether it is from a quality, functional or processing perspective.

Food additives are not used haphazardly in the food industry, they all serve some purpose which can be in the form of making food last longer, improving texture, enhancing flavours which play a crucial role in meeting consumer expectations and the demands of retailers.

Here are some of their main functions:

- **Preserve food**

Without preservatives, some foods simply cannot last, and some products require a longer shelf life so that they are able to be sold in a supermarket where without them, they would spoil quickly which leads to safety risks and food waste. Being able to extend the shelf life of a product is a benefit especially to developing countries. The dosage used for using preservatives is typically very small and is only used whenever possible.

For example, sorbic acid (E200) and sodium benzoate (E211) inhibit mould and bacterial growth, extending shelf life, especially critical in regions with limited refrigeration.

- **Improve the quality and stability of a food - this is where additives such as emulsifiers come in**

Certain foods need additives like emulsifiers, so ingredients don't separate; or humectants, which prevent clumping and keep food moist. Emulsifiers achieve two things, one is the appearance because if something like mayonnaise separates, it is unlikely to sell because of the perception that it is spoiled (it's not, it simply doesn't appear right to consumers and just needs a good shake or stir). That's where emulsifiers like lecithin come in to keep the emulsion intact.

- **Improve the appearance, taste or flavour of a food**

These are additives in the form of colouring, flavours and salts. Typically, these are not functional ingredients and more quality additives to enable a consumer to have a particular sensory experience. Natural and synthetic colours such as curcumin (E100) from turmeric or caramel (E150a-d) make foods visually appealing. Flavour enhancers like monosodium glutamate (MSG, E621) deepen umami notes, elevating taste without excessive salt.

• Aid in the processing of food

These are called processing aids and depending on the product, they will require an additive to ensure that it can be made. Examples of these are enzymes in bread. Enzymes like alpha-amylase (E1100) break down starches in bread-making, improving dough consistency. Processing aids ensure efficiency without lingering in the final product.

• Replace sugars with other ingredients

Products with claims such as 'no added sugar' or 'no sugar added' have replaced sugar with either artificial or natural sweeteners. Sweeteners like steviol glycosides (E960) and erythritol (E968) allow "no added sugar" claims while maintaining sweetness, catering to health-conscious consumers. Monk fruit extract is another popular alternative to sugar and is considered a 'natural' alternative to artificial sweeteners. Monk fruit extract is 100 to 250 times sweeter than sugar and has zero calories and is used in much smaller doses.

• Improve mouthfeel

These additives typically are added to foods where there is an expectation of a certain mouthfeel or texture. Some products like yoghurt have thickeners to give it a mouthfeel or to mimic creaminess. Thickeners like xanthan gum (E415) give yoghurt a creamy texture, while pectin (E440) stabilises jams. Pectin is derived from citrus peels and has been a commonly used additive all around the world. These additives can replicate indulgent textures in healthier formulations and sometimes are required for a product to function properly.

Why do additives seem scary?

Additives 'seem' scary because people don't know what they really are. Additives require rigorous testing to ensure that they are safe for human consumption. Many of these additives have been used for decades or sometimes centuries and used in a plethora of different cultures.

One of the reasons why they seem scary is because of the way they have been portrayed by food marketing. Anything that is an e number or a word that is not commonly used tends to scare away the typical consumer. Or the saying of 'if your grandmother doesn't recognise it, don't eat it'. Here's the reason why, this logic is wrong:

Grandma wouldn't have recognised golden or red kiwifruit and would have rejected it. Food is constantly evolving and changing. Just because something isn't recognised, doesn't mean it's going to harm you. Consumers are not aware of the stringent amount of testing and audits that must be done before a food product can be sold to the public, let alone the supermarket.

Additives get a rebrand

Because of the strong negative sentiment towards additives, product developers and food marketers had to come up with ways to make their ingredients friendlier and more approachable. Sometimes this is called "clean label". What has been done is to simply spell out the additive in a way that is more appealing and understood. Some ingredients with an e number have simply been rebranded into names that are more recognisable and less 'nasty' sounding. For example, instead of colours, an ingredient would say natural black carrot colouring. This makes it seem more recognisable but that black carrot colouring has been

List of additives

Additive type	Function	Example uses	Why it's used
Preservatives	Extends the shelf life of a food product by preventing spoilage by inhibiting bacteria, mould, or yeast growth.	Sodium benzoate (211)Prevents fermentation in sodas and spoilage in acidic condiments. Sulphur dioxide (220) Dried fruits, wine, processed meats. Nisin (234) Dairy products, canned foods	Without preservatives, foods like bread, deli meats, and sauces would spoil within days, increasing waste and foodborne illness risks. Preservatives are used at the lowest effective dose to minimise health risks while maximizing food safety.
Sweeteners	Replace sugar to reduce calories or enhance sweetness.	Stevia glycosides (960) "No-sugar" beverages, yogurts Aspartame (951) Diet sodas, sugar-free gum Sucralose (955) Baked goods, protein bars Erythritol (968) Keto-friendly chocolates, desserts	Sweeteners allow diabetic-friendly and low-calorie products while maintaining taste. Stevia is extracted from stevia leaves, 200–300x sweeter than sugar with zero calories. Sweeteners are safe for most people when consumed within recommended daily limits. While not inherently "healthy", it is used as a tool for reducing added sugar, not a nutritional benefit in itself.
Emulsifiers & Stabilisers	Prevents separation and ingredients mixed together (e.g. oil and water) and improve texture.	Lecithin (322) Chocolate, margarine, ice cream Xanthan gum (415) Gluten-free bread, salad dressings Carrageenan (407) Plant-based milks, custards Pectin (440) Jams, gummy candies	Emulsifiers ensure your peanut butter stays creamy because the oil is not being separated, and your almond milk doesn't separate.

4. The Irresistible Tri Factor

Colourants	Enhance visual appeal or compensate for colour loss during processing.	Curcumin (100) Mustard, curry powders Carmine (120) Yogurts, candies, cosmetics Titanium dioxide (171) White coatings on candies, pastries Anthocyanins (163) Purple/red beverages, confectionery	These are used to heighten or preserve the visual aesthetic of a product.
Antioxidants	Slow oxidation to prevent rancidity in fats or browning in fruits.	Ascorbic acid (300) Fresh-cut fruits, cured meats Tocopherols (307-309) Vegetable oils, cereal bars Citric acid (330) Canned fruits, soft drinks	Oxidation causes "off" flavours and nutrient loss. Antioxidants keep fats in snacks from going stale and preserve vitamin content in processed foods.
Acidity regulators	Adjust pH or add body to foods.	Citric acid (E330) Sour candies, preserved foods Calcium carbonate (E170) Baking powder, fortified plant milks	Controlling the pH or acidity of food means not needing the use of preservatives and it can help maintain taste or inhibit bacterial growth.
Flavour enhancers	Boost savoury (umami) or sweet notes without overpowering. It can help with reducing the amount of salt used in a food product.	Monosodium glutamate (MSG or 621) Instant noodles, soups, snacks Disodium guanylate (627) Potato chips, canned soups	To boost an existing flavour profile, used in some Asian foods and products.
Gelling agents & thickeners	Retain moisture or create gels.	Guar gum (412) Used in ice cream, sauces, baked goods, and gluten-free products to improve texture and prevent ice crystal formation Locust bean gum / Carob bean gum (410) Used in cream cheese, ice cream, and dairy desserts for smoothness and viscosity Xanthan gum (415) Found in salad dressings, sauces, gluten-free baked goods, and beverages for stability and mouthfeel. Carrageenan (407) Extracted from red seaweed, used in dairy products, chocolate milk, and plant-based milks for gelling and thickening.	Also used to modify the creaminess, thickness or firmness of a product and aids in giving a pleasant mouthfeel to the consumer.
Humectants	Helps retain moisture in a product	Glycerin (422) Energy bars, dried fruits	Prevents products from becoming rock hard and clumpy.

around for a long time and had to be rebranded on the packet to make it more palatable to consumers.

The list of additives and what they do

Without certain additives, some foods would not be available or accessible to certain demographics, and it does allow them to preserve, enhance flavours, texture, mouthfeel and appearances of products. Here is a short list of the types of additives and their use cases:

My personal take on additives

I get asked frequently what kind of additives I would avoid. I try when I can to eat whole foods. However, this is not always possible. I do eat the occasional muesli bar which has almost all the different types of additives in some shape or form. Understanding that each additive has a purpose, I personally do not mind if a processed food has flavours, colouring, humectants, acidity regulators and antioxidants as I know how they are made and the doses that are used are so minute that it's very unlikely that they will do something detrimental to you in the long run. When I can, I try to avoid things with preservatives, emulsifiers or thickeners. Preservatives I avoid if I can, I find that they don't work well with my own gut health. That's not to say that it will be like that for other consumers, preservatives are safe, as they are known to kill bacteria, that includes the 'good' bacteria as well.

How food processing works

Nearly all the food we eat has undergone some form of processing, whether it's washing, chopping, or canning. Yet, many consumers have little understanding of what food processing truly entails, partly because proprietary methods are closely guarded by manufacturers (Monteiro et al., 2019). At its core, food processing transforms raw ingredients into safe, convenient, and longer-lasting products while enhancing flavour and texture.

The processing that happens to processed food and ultra processed food is exactly what makes it convenient for consumers, tastier, safer, convenient and longer-lasting.

Food processing comes in many different forms, varieties, industries and has been around for thousands of years. The main difference is that food processing is a strict and controlled activity in every country where food safety is paramount and regardless of the industry, quality control is not an option (Floros et al., 2010).

Food processing in the manufacturing industry involves transforming raw ingredients into food products that are safe, shelf-stable, and convenient for consumers. The methods vary depending on the type of food, desired shelf life, and nutritional goals. Also note that the type of food product doesn't always correlate with the amount of processing it has gone through.

Here's a rundown of the main types of food processing:

1. Primary Processing

The initial step of converting raw agricultural products into a form that can be further processed or consumed. These processes prepare ingredients for further use while maintaining their fundamental properties and the food matrix is intact. This process allows some raw agricultural products to be eaten for direct consumption or further processing.

Examples:

- Cleaning and sorting grains, fruits, and vegetables.

- Milling wheat into flour.

- Shelling nuts or husking corn.

- Slaughtering and dressing meat.

2. Secondary Processing

Transforming primary processed ingredients into edible shelf stable products. This further processing can be in the form of fermentation, drying, heating, freeze-drying, canning etc.

Examples:

- Baking bread from flour.

- Making cheese from milk.

• Producing sausages from meat.

• Canning fruits or vegetables.

3. Tertiary Processing (Value-Added Processing)

Producing highly processed, convenience foods and to extend a food products shelf life. This is usually a combination of different processing techniques where a frozen dinner has freeze-dried ingredients, cut vegetables and is heated before being snap frozen.

Examples:

• Ready-to-eat meals, frozen dinners, and instant noodles.

• Snack foods like chips, cookies, and candies.

• Pre-packaged salads or cut fruits.

Other food processing methods for a specific purpose such as shelf-life extension or texture modification.

4. Thermal Processing

Using heat at high temperatures to preserve food to ensure safety and extend shelf life.

Methods:

• Pasteurisation: Heating to kill pathogens (e.g., milk, juices).

- Sterilisation: High-temperature treatment to eliminate all microorganisms (e.g., canned goods).

- Blanching: Briefly boiling vegetables before freezing.

- Canning: Sealing food in airtight containers and heating.

5. Dehydration

Removing water from food to inhibit microbial growth which extends its shelf life, reduces its weight and preserves some nutrients.

Methods:

- Sun drying (e.g., raisins, tomatoes).

- Spray drying (e.g., milk powder, coffee).

- Freeze drying (e.g., instant coffee, camping foods).

6. Freezing

Lowering the temperature of food to preserve its food matrix and nutritional value.

Methods:

- Flash freezing (e.g., frozen vegetables, seafood).

- Blast freezing (e.g., meat, prepared meals).

7. Fermentation

Using microorganisms (bacteria, yeast, or moulds) to alter food properties such as enhancing flavour, texture and nutritional value or preserve food.

Examples:

- Yoghurt, cheese, and kefir from milk.

- Beer, wine, and sake from grains or fruits.

- Sauerkraut, kimchi, and soy sauce from vegetables or soybeans.

8. Chemical Preservation

Adding chemicals to inhibit spoilage or microbial growth, change the sensory properties and maintain quality over time.

Examples:

- Salt curing (e.g., bacon, fish).

- Sugar preservation (e.g., jams, jellies).

- Adding preservatives like sodium benzoate or sulphites.

9. Mechanical Processing

Physically altering the structure of food which can come in different shapes, forms and intensities usually to either improve texture, consistency or usability.

Examples:

- Grinding, chopping, or slicing (e.g., minced meat, diced vegetables).

- Extrusion (e.g., pasta, breakfast cereals).

- Homogenisation (e.g., milk, sauces).

10. Irradiation

Exposing food to ionising radiation to kill pathogens which helps ensure safety and extends its shelf life.

Examples:

- Treating spices, herbs, and certain fruits so they can last longer without affecting flavour.

11. Aseptic Processing

Sterilising food and packaging separately, then combining them in a sterile environment. Or sometimes the food is sterilised inside specially created packaging that can be specialised with the food which helps extend shelf life and preserves freshness without the need for refrigeration.

Examples:

- Shelf stable containers or packaging for juices and milk that allow them to be stored in ambient temperatures by using a special type of proprietary packaging.

12. High-Pressure Processing (HPP)

Using high pressure to kill pathogens without heat that helps maintain nutritional quality, extends shelf life and maintains freshness.

Examples:

- Cold-pressed juices, deli meats, and guacamole.

13. Extrusion

A form of mechanical processing which involves forcing food through a shaped die under high pressure and temperature to create specific shapes and textures.

Examples:

- Extruded snacks like puffs, swirls and chips.

- Breakfast cereals and pet food.

14. Packaging

Protecting food from contamination and extending shelf life. Some processed foods require multiple packaging steps, depending on customer requirements. Packaging is important to ensure safety, shelf life and convenience.

Methods:

- Vacuum packaging (e.g., cured meats, cheese).

- Modified atmosphere packaging (e.g., salads, fresh meat).

- Aseptic packaging (e.g., milk, soups) where the food is essentially cooked in the packaging and has a long shelf life.

15. Novel and Emerging Technologies

Some food companies deploy new types of technologies in their process that allow them to manipulate or extract certain compounds from foods to differentiate their products from the competition.

- Pulsed Electric Field (PEF): Disrupts microbial cells without heat.

- Ultrasound: Enhances extraction and preservation.

- Cold Plasma: Kills pathogens on surfaces.

Food processing is in essence, large scale cooking except there are teams of people making the products day in and out. The methods that we use for cooking which can include heating, slicing, cutting, pouring, mixing etc are all food processing, however the difference is that we don't call home made food, processed food.

Here's the thing, whatever you call it, in principle homemade food is also processed food. It goes through the same processing as it would in a factory except, it's in your own home and the reason it FEELS like store-bought food is processed food is primarily because you didn't make it, you purchased it.

Processed food is already in a state that your body can break down more easily, hence why when you eat a chocolate or muesli bar, you'll get a sugar rush more quickly compared to eating oats by itself. The real distinction lies in the level of transformation and convenience, now that we start to see through the fear mongering and the marketing, start to consider the different types of innovation behind each food product and how it can be of benefit or detrimental to you.

So how do some foods without preservatives, emulsifiers last longer?

This is where the real food science and food technology comes in. Each industry has a unique way of utilising processing to give a different result that means it relies less on the dependence of additives. The processing can be a combination of the above techniques or a specialisation in that one technique.

An example of this is spray drying where milk is dehydrated and turned into a powder that allows it to last longer by extracting the water and moisture from it, allows it to be used in many different applications, more easily transported and last longer.

It is easy to assume as a consumer that if a product is different from its original state that it has been altered with CHEMICALS when no such thing has happened. This is a misconception amongst processed foods, if any such additives are used and remain in the product, the food manufacturer MUST declare on the pack. There is no way around this, it must be done due to legislation and regulatory measures in places.

What's the deal with emulsifiers?

Emulsifiers are now the new bad guy, but the thing is, they've been around even before processed food was called processed food.

Why are they the new bad guy? There must always be a new 'baddie', thanks to popular culture. There have been recent studies that put emulsifiers in a bad light where there have been reports where there is a link with emulsifier consumption and gut inflammation and cardiovascular disease (Sellem et al., 2023). However, those studies are still inconclusive and evidence in humans of this correlation is still very limited.

Emulsifiers basically help two different types of compounds, typically liquids that don't usually mix to be able to be mixed into one cohesive 'emulsion'. If you put water and oil together, they want to separate. Emulsifiers help them mix together. These are commonly used in ultra processed foods such as peanut butter, hazelnut spread, ice cream, cream-like sauces, biscuits, chocolate.

The classic version of an emulsifier is the egg. Eggs are great emulsifiers because they can help combine different ingredients together. Eggs contain a naturally occurring phospholipid (this is a chemical called lecithin). Eggs aren't always used because they are expensive as an ingredient, some products need to be vegan, and they don't give the same precision or shelf stability compared to an industrial emulsifier. When it comes to emulsifiers and other additives, the dosage and quantities used in food products are usually minimal which are deemed by regulatory bodies to be safe at typical consumption levels (EFSA, 2017). To achieve the desired property for that food product, it is in the food manufacturers' best interest not to overengineer a product.

If you feel that you want to avoid emulsifiers because it is associated with UPF, that's a valid choice. However, demonising them oversimplifies a nuanced issue. Remember that emulsifiers have been around for a lot longer than we realise and it is still inconclusive and almost impossible to determine if emulsifiers are a causal factor in causing things such as cardiovascular disease or gut inflammation. More research is needed to determine if emulsifiers are causal or merely correlative in health risks.

Sensory Science

How do big food companies know when a food product is going to perform well? Is it just an agreement of the leadership team with their expensive opinions and whether they like the product that determines if it will go to the market? Not quite.

This is where sensory science comes in. Sensory science is a specialist field of food technology where the aspects of food such as its appearance, aroma, taste, texture and sound are measured and how it contributes to your sensory experience as a consumer (Lawless & Heymann, 2010).

There is a misconception that food companies measure the dopamine release of a product to determine consumer addiction or purchasing behaviour. This is not the case, measuring such neurological responses like dopamine releases is expensive and unnecessary (Berridge & Kringelbach, 2015).

Sensory science involves creating, measuring, analysing, and interpreting reactions to these sensory experiences. This science also develops methods to determine whether specific levels of stimuli (like flavours or textures) can be detected and whether differences between them can be noticed. The act of conducting such studies is called sensory evaluation. This is especially important in quality control and auditing programs, where consistency is key. For example, it ensures that a product's flavour stays consistent with consumer expectations, that packaging is secure but easy to open, or that potato chips stay crisp throughout their shelf life.

How do sensory evaluations work?

Trained panels, which act like human measuring tools, are often used to detect deviations from a set standard. In some cases, machines can also perform these measurements. These are usually for textural properties like the crunchiness of a chip.

The panels in big food companies usually consist of internal staff who are typically trained to detect the variations in the five basic tastes which are: sweet, sour, salty, bitter and umami. They would then be trained into the specific characteristics of that product (e.g. For milk products, it would be creaminess).

Another common application of sensory science is when a product's ingredients or manufacturing process needs to change. In such cases, manufacturers use sensory tools to ensure that customers don't notice any difference between the old and new versions. These tools can also help identify ways to improve a product to make it more appealing to consumers. This might involve using both trained panels and consumer panels to gather insights and feedback.

How is sensory science or quality control implemented in the food industry?

The food industry wants to ensure that you as a consumer will continue buying the product.

So as a consumer, you wouldn't know about sensory science unless you have worked in the field. Sensory science is used as a tool to ensure that the quality of the food product is to the expectation of the product. Food companies prioritise consistency to retain consumer trust. Product developers taste numerous prototypes before finalising a product, where they usually have to conduct many trials and prototypes before they release their product. Consumers only taste the final product, whereas food product development technologists would have tasted numerous samples to get to the point where it is actually acceptable to the public.

Because everyone has tastebuds that are different from one another, there is no such thing as the 'best' tasting product. This is going to be subjective for every food category possible.

So how does a food product become acceptable to the public? The answer is statistics. It is risky for a food business to be reliant on just a few people to determine whether a food product is palatable. Typically, a food technologist would make sure that the food product is up to their standard before it is presented further internally. Usually, a marketing person and someone in the leadership team will taste different samples and choose one that they collectively feel will work. However, this is not always the case and can mean there is bias for certain taste profiles that are skewed to a group of individuals.

So, when a company needs to make a call for a food product, they must recruit a statistically significant number of people to make up a sensory panel which is usually 30 to 50 people, these can be either internal or external people. But for bigger food businesses, they would recruit a larger internal pool, and this makes it cheaper. This will help food businesses not rely on specific individuals to decide whether a food product is deemed 'acceptable' to the market.

4. The Irresistible Tri Factor

For small food businesses, sometimes they would test this on a small select focus group and get feedback from their target consumers, also called a consumer panel. Such focus groups can be a great way to get unbiased feedback and can prevent most food product launches from becoming a disaster.

For larger food businesses and if they are well resourced, typically corporate, they would have a dedicated sensory team working alongside the quality and product development teams to ensure that the products created are of the standard that their brand and consumers expect.

Sensory science is used for both existing and new food products. If there is a change in an ingredient like a different form, supplier or dosage while there aren't any other changes to that product, then sensory science is used to test whether there is a statistically significant difference that a consumer could pick up. If, for example, an ingredient's supplier has changed, then there is no need to change the packaging. Instead, the company might deploy a sensory session to evaluate whether it's different from the base ingredient. As a consumer, this is something you might not notice. Typically, if there is a statistically significant change, then the dosage to change that ingredient would be done in small doses over time so that the change in the sensory experience isn't so drastic that a typical consumer wouldn't be able to experience or detect it.

Supertaster

Supertasters are individuals who can taste more bitter notes than most people. This is a genetic variation and most commonly found among women.

The difference between a normal human and a supertaster human is the number of tastebuds on the tongue. Supertasters have about ten times more fungiform papillae (taste buds) on their tongues. This heightened sensitivity is primarily linked to a genetic variation in the TAS2R38 gene, which influences bitter taste perception (Hayes et al., 2011).

Supertasters make up about a quarter of the population, with notable genetic, gender, and ethnic differences. Their heightened taste sensitivity influences dietary habits, health outcomes, and even beverage preferences. Understanding these patterns can help in personalised nutrition and food industry applications. Women are more likely to be supertasters (about 35%) than men (15%) (Duffy et al., 2004).

Typically, supertasters are sensitive to bitter foods such as coffee, broccoli, dry red wines. The best way to know if you're a supertaster is to take a PROP test. A PROP test is a strip of paper that has a bitter compound on it and when placed on the tongue, a supertaster will be able to detect it straight away while an average or non-taster will not be able to detect bitter notes on the piece of paper.

4. The Irresistible Tri Factor

It's quite easy to find out if you're a supertaster, if you don't want to do a prop test.

Simply drink black coffee and if it's too bitter for you then you're most likely a supertaster. Otherwise, you can get some blue dye and put one drop on your tongue. Take a picture of your tongue and count how many papillae are on your tongue and do this with a friend or partner and do a comparison.

Here is how you'll know you're a supertaster:

Average person: ~100-150 taste buds/cm².

Supertaster: ~150-200+ taste buds/cm².

Non-taster: ~50-100 taste buds/cm².

There are no real advantages to being a supertaster other than finding bitter, sweet, salty, and spicy flavours more intense than others. It is worth noting that being a supertaster means that you can pay more attention to flavours than your average or non-taster.

I am a super taster myself, and I found this out when I did the prop test in university. My tongue was so sensitive that I couldn't even put the prop paper on my tongue as I could already sense the bitterness when it was close to my mouth. Imagine drinking the most bitter coffee in the world times 1000, that's what the prop test tastes like to a supertaster. For me, I'm not a fan of bitter foods like liquorice, black coffee or things like sour lollies and carbonated water.

From a sensory science perspective, for food technologists it is important to know who a supertaster is on your panel as this could either skew or help your results.

Conclusion: The Irresistible Tri Factor

I still love eating salt and vinegar chips and dark chocolate. I used to love white chocolate and there was a period in my life where I would eat this every single day. It was my way of dealing with stress. I called it my kryptonite, because it reminds me of childhood, but it was probably killing me slowly. I realised that I could not stop eating, and that it was getting to a point where I was turning quite tubby. I found that it was eating into my limited budget and, I was not eating properly. My blood sugar started to spike, and I was a little scared that I was going to get diabetes at a very young age.

I realised that white chocolate does have high amounts of sugar and fat and which contributed to it being irresistible. During my studies, it was a challenge to keep the food you like most in your mouth for as long as possible before ingesting it. So, when I did that with white chocolate, I had to stop and feel how the chocolate melted in my mouth. I could feel the sugar slowly getting to my tongue. I quickly realised that it was far too sweet for me when I slowed down my eating. As if my brain realised, I don't want to eat this as often when I wasn't eating it so quickly. Since then, I've taken my time to eat those irresistible treats and not devour it all at once. It makes me appreciate food more in general. So, I ask you, the reader, to time yourself eating your kryptonite, give yourself 35 seconds to really chew, bite and observe the different sensations.

In conclusion, being aware of the irresistible combination is the first step towards a healthier change. Fat, sugar and salt (FSS) combined with mouthfeel, textures that appeal to the primitive brain are exactly what get you addicted, prioritising taste hits at the expense of your health. The FSS combination will continue to be used to keep you hooked and addicted to certain processed foods and ultra processed foods. In conjunction with the understanding of how the Marketing Tri Factor in the next chapter is used, you can see why it is hard for consumers to move away from processed foods or ultra processed foods. It may take awhile to make a shift in habits however the next time you're in the supermarket, look out for the FSS combination.

🔍 Food detectives shop smarter tip!

Have a look at the following in the nutritional information panel:

Saturated fat – how much of this is coming from actual fat sources, oil? Is this part of the ingredients inherent to the food matrix or is it coming from an additional source like oil? Is this contributing towards the profile of the product?

Sugars – look out for if there are any added sugars, natural sugars occurring from the products inherent nature (milk for example has some naturally occurring sugars)

Salt – how much of this is contributing to your overall salt intake?

For the fat, sugar, and salt, pay attention to the 100g section of the nutritional panel to see how much it is contributing to the product as an overall percentage. If it has more than 20-40% in fat, 20% in sugar, and or 500mg in sodium total, reconsider getting a healthier alternative.

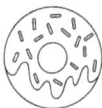

5. The Marketing Tri Factor

Everything that is sold needs some form of marketing. This can come in the form of its branding, logo, packaging, advertising etc.

Marketing is a necessary evil and especially for the food industry where companies need to sell processed food.

As a consumer, you need to stay ignorant because the food industry and its marketing department want it that way. When you're an ignorant and compliant consumer, it is easier to sell to you.

The less that you're relying on due diligence and checking labels the better for the marketing teams as it makes their job easier.

Here's how to be a good ignorant consumer:

- Trust the brands and its logos blindly

- Don't read the labels, nutrition information panels, or where it comes from

- Only read the claims on the front of the packaging

- Buy things on impulse

5. The Marketing Tri Factor

- Rely on your nostalgia for a good time

- Believe that brands determine the quality of a product

- Believe that packaging determines the product quality

- Believe a marketing claim when it says it is natural, real, and has no nasties

- Believe that any "no added sugar" product is better for you

Unfortunately for marketing people, this book is meant to give consumers the awareness to look past the marketing fluff and puff. On the other hand, it also offers an opportunity to be more transparent and hold their food marketing accountable for dubious claims.

The Marketing Tri Factor consists of 3 factors which are the 3 C's:

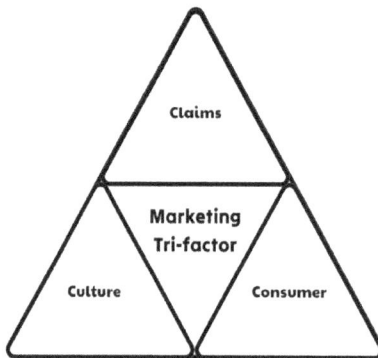

Claims – Almost all food products have either a claim on the packaging or some copy. These are things that will help sell a product and they are a food marketers' tool to get a consumer over the purchasing line. I'll cover how claims and copy are used in ways that a consumer doesn't realise they are being manipulated into purchasing a product.

Culture – Food and culture go hand in hand. When it comes to processed food, it is a little different, our lifestyles also come into play when it comes to processed food. We will cover what are the factors and context that will determine whether or not you will purchase a food product ranging from your age, cultural background, upbringing, stage of life and budget. Also, nostalgia is a part of how we are marketed to with food that reminds us of a time from our childhood that is used to get consumers to purchase food products.

Consumer – Marketing's objective is to convince consumers to buy food products when making a split-second decision. How consumers are viewed by food marketing and the food industry is not how the consumers view themselves. There is a disconnect between consumers, food marketing and the food industry. This disconnect is what helps consumers have a distorted perspective of the food industry which works in marketing's favour. However, this means there is a lack of transparency and trust.

How Food Marketers view consumers

If you look at any food marketing words on processed food packaging, the vocabulary isn't complex. It is typically direct, descriptive and full of words that promise the world. Because processed food cannot speak to its consumer directly and the packaging must be printed on, the wording on it must appeal to the masses.

The masses mean most people, who the food marketers assume have some primary school level of English. Food marketers often assume a baseline literacy level equivalent to that of a 12-year-old, ensuring accessibility for consumers with varying education levels (Harris et al., 2009). Food marketers must assume that their consumers are able to read but perhaps haven't finished high school to ensure that the message they want to relay about the product will be understood and resonate with them. Since these products cannot communicate directly with consumers and must appeal to a mass audience, the language used is deliberately uncomplicated. This strategy aligns with what linguists' term "consumer-grade simplicity," where messaging avoids complexity to maximise comprehension and emotional resonance (Scrinis, 2013).

Certain terms function as "health halos," creating a perception of benefit that may not be substantiated (Andrews et al., 2011). This tactic reflects what scholars describe as "nutritional puffery", exaggerated claims that exploit regulatory loopholes in food labelling (Hieke et al., 2016).

Words like "superfood," despite lacking a standardized legal or scientific definition, are strategically deployed to imply superior nutritional value, capitalizing on consumer desires for health and wellness (Moodie et al., 2013).

Food marketing relies on simple, persuasive language designed to appeal to broad consumer demographics. Processed food marketing typically employs direct, descriptive, and hyperbolic claims on the front of the pack, such as "energy-boosting", "guilt-free" or "farm-fresh" to capture attention and promise exaggerated benefits (Nestle, 2018).

Ultimately, food marketing operates on the premise that consumers are not just purchasing a product but some form of an aspirational identity, whether that's health-consciousness, convenience, or indulgence (Pollan, 2008). By leveraging simplified language, cultural trends, and ambiguous buzzwords, marketers construct narratives that resonate emotionally rather than inform rationally (Elliott, 2012).

What determines what food products you buy: budget, how you buy a food product (lifestyle, health, stage in life, budget, location, culture, occasion, time, values etc)

Food is a BIG part of our lives.

Food is inescapable. From the moment we're born, we're bound to it, not by choice, but by biology. We cannot escape it. We didn't get to choose to eat food. It is what nature simply intended for all life that it requires some kind of nutrients to survive, to have energy and stay alive. It's not just sustenance; it's culture, identity, comfort, and survival. Yet, somewhere along the way, food became more than just nourishment.

It became an industry, a marketing battleground, a political issue, and a mirror reflecting our values, fears, and desires.

There are a plethora of reasons and simply put it's going to be different for everyone individually, holistically and as a society.

If you're reading this, you might be wondering: How did we get here? Why do we rely so heavily on processed foods? How is it that we're so reliant on processed foods? Why are we so unhealthy? Why do some of us struggle to eat well, while others don't think twice about what they toss into their carts?

The answer isn't simple. It's a tangled web of personal circumstances, societal pressures, economic realities, and biological impulses. What drives one person to buy organic kale might push another toward a frozen pizza. And neither choice exists in a vacuum, it's shaped by budget, lifestyle, culture, time, values, and even the subtle psychology of packaging.

When you're a consumer, without knowing, you have been prescribed a way of purchasing your food which suits your current aspirational identity. You won't be known to the food marketing department personally unless you actually work with them. However, it's their job to make sure that you do feel connected. In essence it is a one-sided relationship. The food marketing and product developers get to see your side of the room, like a one-sided mirror, the consumers often just see a reflection of themselves in their food without ever knowing what is happening on the other side.

So, what really determines how we buy food?

Budget/Price

The price of a food product is one of the main drivers of whether a consumer will buy a product or not.

At the time of writing this book, the cost of living and inflation has caused many consumers to be more wary of how much their everyday groceries cost.

Your grocery budget will determine what type of products you will buy, where you will buy them, and on what occasion and how often you will use them.

There is a common misconception that if something is cheaper than it means it is lower quality which is not entirely true. The quality of a product is not always determined by its price; however, products that use higher quality ingredients are typically priced at a higher level.

Sometimes a higher priced product is also used as a marketing tool for promotional purposes.

5. The Marketing Tri Factor

As a consumer, you're looking for food products that are deemed 'reasonably priced'. Reasonably priced means that you're not spending something excessive like 10 dollars for a bag of oats or falling into the discount trap of "Buy one, get one free". These deals encourage over-purchasing, often leading to food waste, yet they're irresistible because they feel like smart shopping (Haws & Bearden, 2006).

Some supermarkets provide a price cost of a product when it is per kg and in the packaging size it is in and that gives an idea to the consumer what the actual cost is.

But price isn't always an indicator of quality. A branded bag of oats might not be inherently better than a bag of private label oats sometimes, you're paying for branding, packaging, or perceived prestige. Supermarkets know this, which is why unit pricing (cost per 100g or kg) is a small but powerful tool for savvy shoppers. Yet, even then, psychological pricing tricks like "99-cent endings" or "limited-time discounts" can override logic (Kahneman, 2011).

Money talks, especially at the grocery store. For most people, price is the ultimate decider. Inflation, rising costs of living, and economic instability force consumers to make trade-offs. A family on a tight budget might prioritise filling their cart over premium ingredients, while others might splurge on organic produce or artisanal products as a form of self-care or status signalling.

It is a quality myth that many assume expensive equals better, but that's not always true. An organic avocado may seem more nutritionally superior to a non-organic conventional avocado with its premium pricing, yet it may not be entirely true that it is healthier.

Lifestyle

Your lifestyle will determine how you buy a product and the brands that you purchase, how often you're purchasing them, how it fits into your work, family and living situation.

If you're a consumer that goes to the gym, you might be more conscious of ensuring that you're purchasing products with more protein content.

If you're a consumer that has young children, you may have purchased a tub of yoghurt just because it's got a picture of a cartoon dog on it that your children love and wouldn't eat it otherwise.

If you're a consumer that is time poor and want products that will be convenient and save you time, products such as premade meals, frozen vegetables and yoghurt pouches might appeal.

Lifestyle isn't just about convenience; it's about identity. What we buy reinforces who we are, or who we want to be (Belk, 1988).

Health/Allergies

Anyone with food allergies, intolerances or living with them is extra vigilant when it comes to purchasing the types of products they consume. Anyone with a strong food allergy will always look out for the allergen statements and read the ingredients list to ensure they won't purchase anything that may cause them potential harm or an uncomfortable stomach.

For those with food allergies, intolerances, or chronic conditions, shopping isn't just a chore, it's a minefield. Gluten-free, dairy-free, nut-free, these aren't trends but are becoming sought after necessities. Every label is scrutinised, every "may contain" warning analysed.

Meanwhile, the rise of functional foods (probiotic yoghurts, vitamin-enriched waters) caters to those chasing wellness. But here's the catch: many "healthy" claims are strategically vague. (Nestle, 2018).

Stage in life

Your stage in life will be a big factor in the types of products you buy. When you're younger, you're probably wanting to buy more energy drinks as it is something that you feel that you need.

It could be that you are looking for products that are low carb because you're on a diet.

Your age and life phase dictate your cravings, and your constraints. Here are some basic stages of life profiles (as a very generalised guide):

Teens & Young Adults: Drawn to energy drinks, instant noodles, and fast food, fuel for late nights and tight budgets. This also applies to adults who are not confident cooking at home, too time poor or enjoy the convenience of purchasing and not cleaning dishes.

New Parents: Shift toward convenience (pureed pouches, pre-cut fruit), snack bars for stroller emergencies and "kid-approved" branding.

Older Adults: May prioritise heart-healthy options (low-sodium soups) or nostalgic comfort foods (classic cereal brands).

Food preferences evolve, but marketers know this, and they target us accordingly. Food companies segment products by life stage, from toddler snacks to senior meal replacements and its marketing messaging and presentation will show this.

Location

Where you are based in the world, country, locally and the socio-economic area where you do your shopping will determine the products that you buy. In low-income urban areas, fresh produce is scarce, leaving fast food and processed meals as the default (Walker et al., 2010).

This will also determine the price of something, and if it's in your locale then you would have more of it than other places. Some countries such as Italy will predominately have tomato and lemon as fresh produce and incorporated into other processed food products.

5. The Marketing Tri Factor

Culture

Your culture in which you are brought up in and where you are located will determine the types of food products you buy and also the cultural awareness that you have is going to determine if you're willing to buy different types of food products from a different culture from yours. Culture runs deeper than just availability, it's about tradition, memory, and belonging. A second-generation immigrant might seek out nostalgic flavours from their parents' homeland, while others might experiment with global cuisines as a form of culinary tourism (Appadurai, 1996).

Occasion

If there are specific types of occasions that are coming up or products that have some kind of emotional connection such as birthdays, then those products will be purchased. Also, some products are only sold during specific parts of the year such as Easter, Christmas, National days in which they would typically be purchased. Food is emotional. Birthdays demand cake. Christmas calls for gingerbread. Heartbreak? Ice cream.

Seasonal marketing exploits this brilliantly, think Cadbury Creme Eggs at Easter or fruit cake during Christmas. These products are more than just food; they're rituals (Douglas & Isherwood, 1979).

Time/Convenience

For consumers that are time poor, they might be purchasing products that are easy to consume, on the go, prepackaged and are typically a single serve.

Or they are an ingredient that has already been processed such as being cut, diced, shredded etc so it's convenient for cooking.

The rise of pre-cut fruit, microwave meals, and protein bars isn't laziness, it's about getting it done efficiently. Single-serving packaging, grab-and-go snacks, and meal delivery kits cater to those who are too busy to cook, but too health-conscious to ignore nutrition entirely.

Values

Your values determine how you purchase products; it could be that you want to support locally made food products, you don't want to buy caged eggs, you want to purchase products that have recyclable packaging.

For example:

Ethical concerns: Free-range eggs, Fair Trade coffee, or boycotts of brands with poor labour practices.

Environmental impact: Reusable packaging, plant-based meats, or "ugly" produce to reduce waste.

Political Statements: Buying local to support small farms or avoiding certain brands due to corporate activism.

The paradox is that ethical or seemingly ethical products are often pricier, making them inaccessible to low-income shoppers. These choices aren't just about taste, they are also about belief systems (Johnston & Szabo, 2011).

5. The Marketing Tri Factor

Presentation

How a product is presented is a major factor in whether a food product is being purchased, to the brand, packaging, messaging, where it sits on the shelf and if you find the product appealing from an aesthetic point of view. Presentation of many products is the reason why there are many different types of marketing, packaging and price points for what is essentially the same product.

The colours and shelf placement of a food product are used to lure you in as a consumer:

Colour Psychology: Green = natural, red = indulgent, black = premium (Ampuero & Vila, 2006).

Shelf Placement: Eye-level products sell 35% more than bottom-shelf ones (Chandon et al., 2009).

"Premium" Aesthetics: Matte finishes (these typically cost more for the packaging, and you the consumer will pay for it), minimalist fonts, and earthy tones signal "artisanal" quality, even if the product is mass-produced.

There are many so-called "luxury" foods that are identical or close to their cheaper counterparts, they are just packaged and marketed differently.

Preferences and Habits

Your preferences of what you like and don't like ultimately will determine whether you buy a food product or not. Sometimes a food product could be something that you eat regularly as a snack and enjoy. These preferences for food can change over time for some people whilst for others this can remain the same for their entire life. Your habits and lifestyle determine what you're going to buy. Habits such as whether you eat breakfast or not, if you like to drink coffee, the type of milk you have with your tea or coffee. All these small little details in your habits are built up over time. Most grocery decisions are unconscious routines:

Brand Loyalty: You buy the same cereal every week because it's familiar, not because it's the best.

Sensory Triggers: The smell of fresh bread or samples can override rational choices.

The "Default" Effect: If you always grab almond milk, you'll keep doing so unless something disrupts the habit (Neal et al., 2011).

Breaking habits is a challenge and requires active effort, which is why brands fight so hard to become your automatic choice.

Education

Your education and awareness of food and nutrition also play a part in the types of food products you will buy. Perhaps you know the different types of probiotic strains, the antioxidant levels of chocolate or that you go for something with no artificial sweeteners.

The basics of Food Marketing

Food marketing is a combination of how the branding, logo, claims, sexy advertising, romance copy, country of origin, and awards will convince a consumer that they only need to see a product without them seeing the ingredients list.

Dissecting a food product: Packaging and Marketing

How to dissect a food product from the packaging and the marketing?

Take any food product that you have in your pantry or shelf.

As a food technologist, we would do this to 'size up' and analyse our competitors. Typically, this exercise was called a competitor analysis. Instead of just looking at it from a marketing perspective, we'd also look at it from a product and packaging perspective too.

For any product, here are the things that we investigate and break down:

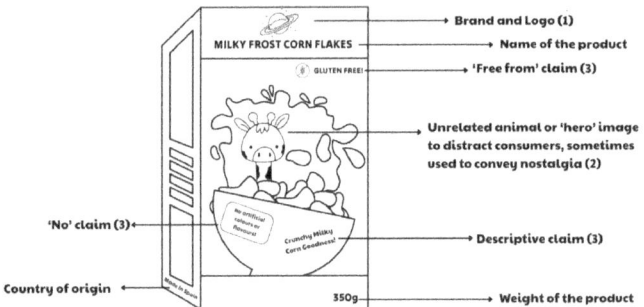

Product basics

Category

Food and beverages have different types of categories, and they will have subcategories. Depending on the retailer or the kind of consumer you are, you will see these very differently. Some consumers will gauge food categories based on the brand and not question if there is a subcategory.

Let's take, for example, yoghurt. This is a broad category. Inside the yoghurt category you'd have subcategories that can include probiotics, lactose free, sugar free, luxury. Look at any food category in the supermarket and you'll see different subcategories. The example in the picture above would be in the cereal category and would be then subcategorised as a budget product assuming it is private label (this will be explained later).

Typically, the subcategories are split between the following (Note: Every company and agency does this slightly differently, depending on the industry):

- Budget
- Mainstream
- Premium

Budget categories are typically the food, beverages where there is minimal marketing and branding effort. Sometimes these are the 3rd party manufactured products for supermarkets where it is cheaper, usually with less or different ingredients compared to the standard mainstream category. These categories are for a specific type of shopper/consumer. The products that wouldn't have a budget category are usually fresh produce and if a consumer wanted to get cheaper produce or reduced to clear/close to expiry date, there are some local supermarkets that will sell those at a heavily discounted price which can include the mainstream and premium categories.

There are local supermarkets in some countries where failed or poorly performing products are sold so the supplier must sell them at a reduced cost to get rid of the inventory. Typically, this is a last resort. However, for consumers looking to save money, this is a great alternative.

The mainstream category is where there is more marketing/branding effort behind pushing the product and this is where most products will sit. They will have something that will differentiate themselves from the rest of the products in their category or subcategory.

These would be your Cadbury, Mars, etc where they are brands recognisable from any supermarket around the world albeit some countries have different versions of these global brands just in their local language.

Premium category is where there are far more marketing and branding put into it and sometimes, they are not always sold in the supermarket. They can be niche products that can be bought at niche luxury stores or online shops. Premium categories are the 'fancier' versions of your mainstream items, think of luxury chocolates that you can't buy from the supermarket, and made from a boutique chocolatier.

Functionally they may do the same (giving you calories) with some slight variations but the perception of how it's presented by its branding makes it stand out from the rest. Each product will taste differently from each company but sometimes there are companies that can just change the packaging of a product/brand differently with the same food product and charge a premium for it.

Also unbeknownst to consumers and even some producers, there are also private label products. Where the product is manufactured by a larger corporation, but its branding is owned by a smaller marketing company or the supermarket.

Company Produced by

The company or organisation that made the food product isn't something that a consumer typically looks at unless they want to make a complaint about the product. However, I think that as a consumer that is reading this book and is more aware, I'd recommend looking at exactly who is making your food.

A quick Google search will tell you everything you need to know. Have a look at the back of a product and see the company details. Every food product needs to provide their company details.

5. The Marketing Tri Factor

Many brands, especially premium ones, will use branding, advertising and logos as a means to disguise who really owns them.

Storage: Ambient, Chilled or Frozen

The storage conditions of a food product are important for both safety and marketing reasons. Mainly for safety reasons, some food products such as fresh milk need to be refrigerated.

The storage conditions for food products are important for food safety and quality. Chilled and frozen products like milk, yoghurt and ice cream will be typically placed at the back of the supermarket so that shoppers must walk past the fresh produce or other products to get to them.

The majority of ultra processed foods have room temperature storage. This is for convenience and that the product itself would have been processed in a way or there will be added preservatives to make it last at room temperatures.

Price

Most consumers will determine if they buy a product by its price. Food products are priced by their ingredients, marketing, packaging, the margins that the supermarkets want (The price of a product is mostly determined by the supermarkets, who take a very large cut from suppliers ranging from 20 to 60%), processing costs, distribution and logistics. Some products will determine cost depending on how a food company can influence retailers with promotions, discounts or favours.

Everyone wants a good deal especially when it comes to groceries. The best way to gauge what works for you, your family and your budget is to know what your non-negotiables are. Is there a product that you must have in your household? Try out different alternatives and find out for yourself, sometimes cheaper alternatives can be better.

Which stores sell the product/Stockists

Food products will have stockists, locations or vendors where they are sold. These aren't on the product itself but sometimes on the product's website. For mainstream supermarket products from global corporations, they won't be there as it's a given that those products will be in a supermarket.

Health star rating

Some countries used a traffic light or number system but essentially these are government initiatives to help consumers choose 'healthier' food products. For the health star rating, the more stars it has (up to 5 stars and it goes up or down in 0.5 increments). These are usually voluntary schemes that a food producer can put on them if they want to. These are meant to be used as guides for consumers who want to make a quick decision on purchasing a food, and to encourage healthier eating. There is a push in the food industry to make the health star rating compulsory. However, there is still debate and discussions on the validity of the scheme and whether the calculations of the star rating are fair and if it makes sense.

Type of packaging

Packaging for food is made so that it can store food safely, can be stacked, portable, lightweight, and easy to use. Now it is a requirement in most supermarkets for packaging materials to be able to be recycled, more on this in later chapters.

Awards

Some food products get awards, and they are displayed on the front of the pack usually. These awards are typically where the producer must pay a fee to enter their product to be able to win by a panel. Not all products enter food awards, and it is not always an indication of the quality of food. This is an exercise that helps a food product get a nice-looking gold or silver badge on its packaging.

Product itself:

Nutritional information - does it show the daily intake column? Displaying the daily intake column is optional by the food manufacturer.

Allergens

Allergens must be shown on all products; this is a legal and mandatory requirement. Not showing allergen information could lead a company to recalling their product, pay a hefty fine, tarnish its brand reputation and even face criminal charges if consumers are harmed.

What the food product is made of

Some food products have simple ingredients whilst others have more than what you'd think. An example of this is Chicken nuggets made with 100% chicken breast. The implication that something made with 100% chicken breast, seems more healthier when in fact, it probably has thickeners, salts, flavour enhancers that would be typical of any chicken nugget. The 100% chicken breast is ONLY for the chicken component and not the entirety of the product itself.

The Role of Branding in Food Marketing

Brand - the brand of a food product is also its company identity, product identity or simply a co-manufactured brand or a store brand (For example a supermarket's brand of biscuits could be called 'Best Selection with 40% chocolate chips').

Brands are a great way for big corporations to disguise their products as if it's a 'local' product amongst the sea of branded food products.

It allows consumers to find the product they remember, recall the sensory experience of what they feel about that product, and associate it with the perceptions that they have of the product.

The brand of a food product will be very important and sometimes it's a big deciding factor if a consumer will buy it. Brands build loyalty with consumers, and it takes years to build trust usually with a good sensory experience, clever marketing and advertising.

Brands sometimes do this with an eye-catching logo so that consumers can recognise their products immediately.

A brand is far more than just a logo or a name: it embodies a company's identity, product positioning, and even consumer perception.

Whether it's a multinational corporation, a private-label product, or a co-manufactured store brand, branding serves as a crucial tool for differentiation in a saturated market (Keller, 2013).

Private label product means that it is manufactured by a third party and then sold under the retailer's own brand name. Private label products are usually created exclusively for the client or retailer, and they set the parameters and standards of what that product should have. For example, there are some fresh milk products that also have private labels (usually for a large supermarket)/third party where they are produced by the same manufacturer (it's the same milk, sometimes cheaper).

For instance, large food conglomerates often employ a strategy known as "brand masking", where they create subsidiary brands designed to appear artisanal, local, or independent, despite being mass-produced (Howard, 2016).

This allows corporations to appeal to niche markets such as organic or farm-to-table consumers, while maintaining economies of scale. The best way to lure consumers away from locally made products is to mimic local branding.

Without strong branding, even a high-quality product like peanut butter would struggle to stand out among nearly identical competitors. Brands function as mental shortcuts for consumers, evoking sensory memories (e.g., taste, texture), emotional associations (e.g., nostalgia, trust), and perceived value (Aaker, 1996). This is why brand loyalty is so powerful for food companies. Once a consumer develops a positive connection with a product, they are more likely to repurchase it, even if cheaper or healthier alternatives exist (Kapferer, 2012).

Logos - A logo is part of a brand, and it makes it easier for consumers to identify goods or services. Logos are memorable, unique, give you an emotional response related to the good or service.

Logos are used everywhere, not just in the food industry. In food businesses, a logo would be featured in its packaging usually on the front of the pack. A logo's typography, colours, style and placement are all part of making it recognisable by its customers.

A logo is more than just a visual mark, it is the face of a brand, a symbol that instantly connects consumers to a product's identity, values, and emotional appeal (Keller, 2013). In the food industry, logos serve as quick identifiers, helping shoppers recognise familiar products in a crowded marketplace, think of the playful swirl of Cadbury's script or the bold red of KitKat. These designs are not arbitrary; they are meticulously crafted to evoke specific feelings such as trust, nostalgia, indulgence, while reinforcing brand loyalty (Aaker, 1996).

While logos are universal across industries, food brands rely on them heavily due to the sensory and emotional nature of consumption. A well-designed logo on packaging acts as a silent salesperson, leveraging:

- Typography – A font can convey tradition (e.g., Coca-Cola's cursive) or modernity (e.g., Beyond Meat's clean sans-serif).

- Colour psychology – Red triggers appetite (McDonald's), green suggests health (Whole Foods), and gold implies premium quality (Lindt) (Singh, 2006).

- Placement & simplicity – The most effective logos are instantly recognisable even in small sizes (e.g., Nike's swoosh), which is why food brands prioritize front-of-pack visibility.

However, logos can also be tools of deception. Some brands use wholesome imagery (e.g., farm landscapes, artisanal scripts) to mask industrialized production (Pollan, 2008).

Marketing copy

In the industry this is also called romance copy. These are usually the text on the back of the product to describe the sensory experience of the product and usually to fill up space, sometimes it might have a story behind it talking about the origins of the product.

What consumers should watch out for

While branding can help consumers identify preferred products, it can also be used to mislead. Here are key red flags to consider:

1. **"Greenwashing" and fake authenticity:** Terms like "natural," "farm-fresh," or "crafted" are often unregulated and used to create a false sense of quality or sustainability (Scrinis, 2013), there will be a section to elaborate on why the term "natural" is more problematic than it seems. Always check for certifications (e.g., Certified Organic, Fair Trade) rather than relying on marketing claims.

2. **Parent company transparency:** Many "small-batch" or "local" brands are actually owned by multinational corporations (e.g., Coca-Cola's Honest Tea, Nestlé's Sweet Earth). Researching parent companies can reveal whether a brand aligns with your values.

3. **Health halo:** Buzzwords like "superfood," "antioxidant-rich," or "protein-packed" can make products seem healthier than they are. Always read the nutrition label rather than trusting front-of-package claims (Nestle, 2018).

4. **Ingredient sourcing & ethical claims:** Brands may highlight one ethical practice (e.g., "cage-free eggs") while ignoring others (e.g., unfair labour practices). Look for third-party audits (e.g., B Corp, Rainforest Alliance) for verification.

5. **Psychological pricing tricks:** "Premium" branding often justifies higher prices without actual quality differences. Comparing unit prices (e.g., cost per gram) helps avoid overpaying for marketing hype (Wansink, 2006).

As a consumer, be aware that the larger the company, the more resources and budget they will have to bring awareness and attention to their products and brands. To start becoming a conscious consumer, you must look beyond branding to assess a product's true value which means: scrutinising ingredients, sourcing, and corporate practices rather than falling for clever packaging or emotional appeals.

Larger food corporations would use endorsements especially sports, athletes or renowned characters from Disney for example to be on their packaging to sell more. These endorsements are expensive so only the big companies can afford to use them for a certain time or promotional period. Certain cereals as an example like to use athletes as a figurehead for their packaging as it helps further their brand and messaging that it is a cereal for athletes.

Lots of small to medium sized businesses are often relying on word of mouth or their own social media pages to get their product known.

> 🔍 **Food detectives shop smarter tip!**
>
> Here are some things to look out for in food marketing and to ask yourself:
>
> **Why do you use this brand?**
> For some consumers like yourself, sometimes we use them because our parents and grandparents use them and it is what we saw working until we are adults. It's best to try different brands of products so you can get a feel of how different the experience is.
>
> **What do you feel when you're using a product with this brand?**
> For some consumers being able to have a brand in their lifestyle is the reason why they purchase in the first place because it makes them feel good, happy or luxurious.
>
> **Are you paying for real value or just the branding?**
> Some products cost more simply because of marketing or shelf position. For basics like flour or baking powder, the brand often doesn't change much. But for products like dark chocolate, different techniques and processes genuinely create different experiences, and the marketing reflects that.

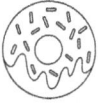

Knowing what is the marketing that is distracting and what is going to be useful

Ultra processed foods have many marketing distractions that can confuse consumers or mislead them into thinking it is healthier than it actually is.

Marketing for any product is essential, so it is appealing to its target consumer. However, some marketing activities and visuals are used as a smokescreen and sometimes are there to distract you from something that they don't want you to see straight away from the product, let's go over some examples of these.

> 🔍 **Food detectives shop smarter tip!**
>
> As a consumer, make sure that you do the following:
>
> Look beyond the logo, always check ingredient lists and certifications rather than trusting a rustic design.
>
> Notice colour manipulation where "healthy" greens or "natural" browns may distract from poor nutritional value.
>
> Recognise brand families: Many logos are variants of large parent corporate companies
>
> Understanding logos and food branding strategies will help you see past the design, how visual cues drive your own purchasing decisions and into what a brand truly represents.

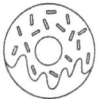

The power of nostalgia and its role in making you purchase food

Nostalgia acts as an emotional anchor, transporting consumers back to simpler, happier times, often childhood. Research shows that nostalgic triggers (e.g., taste, smell, packaging) activate the brain's reward system, releasing dopamine and creating a sense of emotional warmth (Loveland et al., 2010). This explains why adults willingly pay premium prices for:

- Discontinued relaunches (e.g. Dunkaroos in Australia)
- Limited-edition throwbacks (e.g. McDonalds SzeChuan sauce popular from Mulan's animated release followed by a resurgence when mentioned in the Rick & Morty cartoon)
- Reimagined classics (e.g. "Mini" versions of chocolates like Reese's Cups)

Food brands and marketing exploit this by:

- Replicating past sensory experiences (e.g. the crunch of Pringles)

- Using retro branding (e.g. Pepsi's '90s logo revival)

- Partnering with pop culture (e.g. Netflix's Stranger Things x Eggo waffles)

There are several ways how food marketing will utilise nostalgia and weaponise your childhood memories as a form of invisible blackmail to make you purchase their products:

1. The "Remember when?" strategy

Companies reintroduce discontinued products as "limited editions" to create urgency and nostalgia-driven demand.

Example: McDonald's McRib, this was a cult favourite that reappears sporadically, not due to supply issues, but as a marketing tactic (Gabriel, 2019).

2. Generational marketing

Brands target adults who grew up with their products, knowing they'll buy them for their own kids. Example: Coco pops, still used decades later to evoke parental nostalgia (Meyers, 2014).

3. Sensory triggers

Taste and smell are deeply linked to memory. Brands like Nestlé and Hershey's maintain consistent flavours to ensure emotional recall (Herz, 2016).

4. "Shared Nostalgia" in advertising

Commercials often depict family gatherings, school lunches, or holiday traditions to reinforce emotional connections. Example: Coca-Cola's "Summer is here" campaign.

The dark side of nostalgia marketing

While nostalgia can seem like harmless fun, it does have ethical concerns:

Health manipulation: Many nostalgic foods (e.g., Lunchables, Pop-Tarts) are ultra-processed yet marketed as "wholesome" childhood staples. Note that the word "wholesome" is close to the word "whole foods" which mean very different things.

False authenticity: Certain brands profit from nostalgia while cutting ingredient quality.

Exploiting emotional vulnerability: People under stress or feeling lonely are more susceptible to nostalgia-driven purchases (Routledge et al., 2013).

How to consume nostalgia mindfully

If you want to enjoy your childhood nostalgic foods without falling for manipulative marketing, here are a few things you can do:

Nostalgia is a powerful tool that food brands use to foster loyalty, justify premium pricing, and drive impulse purchases. While there's nothing wrong with enjoying a childhood snack for sentimental reasons, consumers should remain aware of how nostalgia is weaponised to override rational decision-making. By understanding these tactics, we can enjoy the past without being controlled by it.

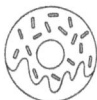

How food claims work

What is a food claim?

Claims are something that you see on the front of the pack and are usually justified by information found on the back of the pack. A food claim on packaging can be a carefully crafted marketing tool designed to influence consumer perception and purchasing decisions. Among the most prominent elements on a package are claims; statements that highlight certain attributes of the product, whether nutritional, ethical, or sensory. These claims are typically displayed on the front of the pack and should, in theory, be substantiated by information on the back. However, the way they are presented, and the language used, can significantly shape consumer interpretation, sometimes blurring the line between factual information and marketing persuasion (Hieke et al., 2016).

There are different types of food claims that are on the pack, let's go through the different categories:

5. The Marketing Tri Factor

- Descriptive claims

- Sensory claims

- Health claims

- Soft ingredient claims

- Country of origin or provenance claims

- Processing claims

Descriptive claims

These are typically the 'romance copy' to describe the product in a nice, descriptive, fluffy way to entice the consumer. It is the text that the majority of people don't read and to fill up space on the back of the pack and to distract the consumer from reading the ingredients, country of origin or the nutritional panel.

Descriptive claims are exactly that, and to avoid any kind of legal implications some descriptive product claims will describe the feeling you get from eating the product. For example, a Coke can mention happiness, chocolates will have words like "decadent", "velvety" etc (Parker, 2017). While some descriptive claims may hold truth (e.g., "slow roasted" for a coffee brand), many fall under puffery, legal exaggeration that consumers are expected to recognise as marketing flair rather than factual promise (FDA, 2021).

Lindt chocolate had a class action lawsuit against them alleging that they had misled consumers into thinking that their chocolate was "expertly crafted with the finest ingredients" when it was found that some of their dark chocolate products were found to have higher-than-allowed amounts of cadmium and lead. The lawsuit claims that the quality and safety of their chocolate was misleading given the presence of those heavy metals and led consumers to believe that it was free from such contaminants. At the time of writing, the court has since denied Lindt's motion to dismiss this lawsuit which highlights the potential that consumers were deceived due to marketing claims.

Sensory experience claims

These are the claims where they are describing the taste, textures, mouthfeel or flavours of the product in a descriptive way. However, these are subjective and not always accurate. These are usually to make the designs less empty and to give a little 'joy' on the packet.

Soft ingredient claims

Soft ingredient claims are when the product highlights a specific feature of an ingredient in the product which has certain "beneficial" properties. Some of these soft ingredient claims can include "Oranges contain Vitamin C", "Blueberries are loaded with antioxidants". These are called soft ingredient claims because it is not about the product that contains the ingredients, only the ingredients, so from a legal point of view and marketing perspective, it is easier to put these on the pack. However, if a product contains only the flavour and not the ingredient itself, it cannot use a soft claim. Because they avoid explicit health promises, they face fewer regulatory hurdles (Nocella & Kennedy, 2012). However, research shows that consumers often misinterpret these claims as endorsements of the product's overall healthfulness (Lähteenmäki, 2013).

Health claims

These are claims about the product's benefits when it is consumed. Unlike soft ingredient claims, health claims explicitly link consumption to a physiological benefit. These are heavily regulated in many regions (e.g., EFSA in Europe, FDA in the U.S.) and must be backed by scientific evidence (EFSA, 2022).

Typically, these claims would be proven with some sort of study or evidence that shows their product provides the benefit. Soft ingredient claims and health claims can sometimes be blurred for the consumer as they can be quite confusing to differentiate. However, it comes down to the wording. If the product says, "Eating two tubs of XYZ yoghurt can help with boosting your immune system" as opposed to "Probiotics help with gut health", the former is a health claim whilst the latter would be a generic soft ingredient claim.

Health claims help a product differentiate itself from the competition and usually they are just general health claims as opposed to specific health claims. Typically, you won't see any food products in western countries where they claim they can cure cancer. This would be illegal.

However, the claim that "yoghurt can help boost your immune system" is often backed by clinical evidence that the food company would have conducted before making such a health claim. The key word choice here is 'can', not 'will' so that the claim does not imply a guarantee of boosting your immune system. Meanwhile, the word 'boosting' implies improving.

Also, many health claims include the caveat along the lines of "as part of a balanced diet" to avoid guaranteeing results. This is a necessary disclaimer, given that few consumers actually follow such diets (Grunert & Wills, 2007). The problem is many people do not know or have a 'balanced diet' and that could look quite different for everyone.

Country of origin or provenance claims

The provenance and locality of a product can be an important claim and feature for a lot of consumers. This is to highlight that you're supporting a local producer/supplier.

However not all 'locally' made products are the same. These are the 'Made in USA' or 'Produced in Australia' claims. However, some products go further than stating it is made in a specific country and actually call out the specific town or region where the product is made.

This is to give the consumer a sense of local pride that the product is made in their hometown.

These are usually done for processed foods where the food matrix hasn't been completely degraded, or its original state is still close to what it looks like in nature e.g. Italian tomatoes.

Some products LOOK locally made but could be produced in another country. These are products where the company is BASED in the local country where it will claim that the product is 100% Australian owned as an example. Or the product is made/packaged in the country but doesn't use any local ingredients.

Studies indicate that origin labelling influences purchasing behaviour, especially when consumers associate certain regions with superior production standards (Van Ittersum et al., 2007).

Processing claims

Processing claims are used to highlight if a processing method has or has not been used (e.g., "slow roasted" for a coffee brand). Some milks use this where they say it is not homogenised or not heat treated to showcase that it has more perceived nutritional value. Processing claims usually are a technological differentiation for certain products which are deemed beneficial to the consumer, with statements like "more nutrients", "no preservatives added" etc.

The other processing claim is the "no preservatives", "no nasties" claim which is to show a particular product hasn't had any specific additives added.

However, these claims can be misleading particularly the "No nasties" claim. This could imply that there are no preservatives, emulsifiers etc however it doesn't necessarily mean it's a better product. The "no nasties" claim is a vague term implying purity but lacking a legal definition, potentially misleading shoppers into believing the product is healthier than its alternatives (Gravely & Fraser, 2018).

You're paying as much for the branding and experience you get as for the product itself. From opening the packaging to putting the food into your mouth, it is all part of the experience. Food with great marketing does more than just highlight the ingredients of the food and highlight the want or need that it satisfies.

Every product you see on a supermarket shelf has a marketing team or person behind the nice fancy uplifting 'romance copy' words on the pack. It is to appeal to your basic wants and needs to make it seem like you're missing out on something, the product may complement your diet or enhance your snack time.

Marketers have a plethora of resources that use psychological techniques that capture consumers' attention.

The majority of consumers, even including myself, are making decisions on a product in less than 3 seconds. Depending on the consumer that you are, the main priorities for a food product are:

5. The Marketing Tri Factor

- Taste

- Price

- Brand

- Convenience

Not always in this order, and it depends on your situation and lifestyle.

Some very effective food marketing is Snickers from Mars. Mars is a global family-owned business which has a large market share of the FMCG (fast moving consumer goods) industry.

One of their slogans is "Always satisfies".

No mention that Snickers contains nougat, peanuts, or caramel.

However, as a consumer, you know that if you eat a Snickers bar, your hunger will be satisfied from those ingredients, and they don't need to be specifically named.

Food marketing can be confusing and sometimes vague on purpose.

For example, you might see "Vegan gummy bears" for sale. Some food companies like to put claims on their packaging to get the PERCEPTION that it is healthier than it is.

The vegan gummy bears can include claims on its packaging that it is all natural and healthy. However, its sugar content is 3 teaspoons or 70g of sugar per 100g. Not exactly healthy but still vegan, and food companies with this kind of marketing are sometimes hoping that consumers make that association between being vegan and being healthy.

Another classic example is Marshmallows. Marshmallows make the claim that they are 99% fat free. However, they have high levels of sugar in them. This is still riding on the belief in the 90s and early 2000s that fat was deemed the devil in food, until sugar was given its spotlight as the villain.

From a food technologist's perspective, sugar is added to foods because it simply adds flavour and taste. It makes a consumer come back and have a repeat purchase which is exactly what a food business wants. However, the industry is moving towards adding less sugar in foods as there is increasing awareness of the detrimental effects that sugar has on the body.

The "No" claims

These are the claims that are on many 'healthy' themed products where the marketing will state there are no additives, preservatives, nasties, artificial colours. These are essentially called negative claims where its omission of certain ingredients make it seem more beneficial.

However, these are typically used on ultra processed foods that still have refined sugars, carbohydrates which are no better for you (more on this later).

The general ingredient claim

The general ingredient claim is typically used for products where there is an ingredient/s that are deemed healthy or beneficial, an example of this would be calling out a blueberry as an ingredient and stating that blueberries are high in antioxidants. However, it doesn't mean that the product itself has high antioxidants, it is simply a way to get a positive association with that product, this kind of claim can be misleading.

The "Limited edition"

Limited editions are usually marketing activities to get consumers excited about a new type of flavour, product or packaging. Limited editions are only for a brief period or for a specific promotion such as win a draw or redeem merchandise. This is making use of FOMO (fear of missing out) and are often used in conjunction with popular franchises to lure consumers to buy food products just because of the association.

The "free from" claims

The 'free from' is very similar to the "No" claims or the negative claims in which a product would say it is 'free from' things such as nasties, additives or certain allergens.

Branding for the sake of differentiation – Private label

Private labels are an industry secret. Not many consumers know about them, however there are some products on the market that are exactly the same, and the only difference is the brand, and slightly different packaging.

Supermarkets have what we call in the industry "private-label" products. These are products that very much mimic branded products, but it has the supermarkets own brand instead. You'll see these in all the major supermarkets. If you live in Australia, Coles has Wellness Road, Woolworths has Woolworths select and Aldi has their own brands for every category.

These private label products are typically cheaper than their branded products. And sometimes, in fact, more often than not, they can be produced by the branded products' manufacturer.

Why do supermarkets do this?

They want to have their own product on their shelves and not someone else's. An example of a popular private label product is Coles Chocolate Chip cookies in Australia. These are delicious chocolate chip cookies that are usually cheaper than your other branded cookies or they will have more cookies for the same price than other brands. Supermarkets do this so they can bring in more profit to their business.

Some food companies can also have the same formulation or a minor tweak of a current product and sell that as a private label product. Unless you work in that food company, it's not so obvious. However, the hint is that if it has the same packaging, nutritional information and ingredients as a branded product then more than likely it is from the same company. Not always the case but that's the easiest way to figure it out.

5. The Marketing Tri Factor

Some food companies don't have strong marketing teams or don't have any marketing at all. Instead, they will rely on marketing companies to market their product, or a marketing company will ask a food company to make their product for them.

In the past few decades, we have seen a slew of 'healthy' foods claiming to be good for you. There was a time when cigarettes were considered 'healthy'!

Healthy foods have different criteria, different meanings for different people. The cycle repeats with new buzzwords. Let's dissect the ever-shifting criteria for "healthy" and expose the myths behind them. The goalposts of "healthy" have moved and changed over time, often with little scientific basis:

1950s–60s: "Low-fat" = healthy (spoiler: replaced with sugar).

1980s–90s: "Cholesterol-free" (ignoring trans fats).

2000s–today: "Organic," "plant-based," "keto-friendly" (often masking ultra-processing).

Research shows these definitions are marketing constructs, not nutrition science (Scrinis, 2013).

For example:

Some "low-fat" yoghurts often contain more sugar than ice cream (Moss, 2013).

"Gluten-free" junk food can be just as unhealthy as regular junk food (Wu et al., 2015).

Now let's have a look at some of the claims that restaurants, cafes, and certain food products use:

- Organic
- Sustainable
- Fresh

Organic

Organic certification: Legally, "organic" requires audits (e.g., USDA, EU Organic Logo) to restrict pesticides/ GMOs (USDA, 2023). Food companies cannot simply use the word organic because they feel their product is better than the competition.

Whilst there's absolutely nothing wrong with foods that are organic, sustainable, or fresh, in fact it should be encouraged, there is a 'healthy halo' effect on these foods. Just because something is labelled organic, sustainable and/or fresh doesn't necessarily mean it's "healthy".

You can have organic potatoes that are baked and then drizzled with organic mayonnaise, it will be the same caloric value that you get from a non-organic potato with non-organic mayonnaise. However, some will opt for the organic potato because it's perceived to be healthier.

To state that a food is organic does require certification in most countries. Food companies cannot simply state that their food is organic, they must be able to prove that it is. Any symbol that carries an Organic logo usually costs the business money to be able to display and the business must substantiate through certification that their product is organic through ongoing audits, and this cost is passed onto the consumer.

Organic sugar is still sugar. Organic fries are still fries. Calories and metabolic effects don't vanish because a food is organic (Dangour et al., 2009).

Sustainable

There isn't a regulated definition for the word 'sustainable' unlike "organic," any brand can claim their product is "sustainable" without proof (FAO, 2021).

Example: "Sustainable" palm oil may still drive deforestation (Meijaard et al., 2020).

At the time of writing this book, sustainable can still be used as a marketing claim and there is no organisation that issues sustainable food logos or certifications.

Fresh

This is a psychological trick where the word "fresh" evokes farm-to-table imagery, but many "fresh" foods are treated to preserve appearance (e.g., supermarket "fresh" bread often contains dough conditioners) (Parker, 2020).

Organic potato chips vs. regular: Same calories, same fat, same blood sugar spike.

"Antioxidant-rich" soda: A sprinkle of vitamin E doesn't offset 40g of sugar (Cohen, 2022).

What does factor into what is healthy is whether it gives your body energy, immunity (antioxidants, vitamins), good fat, protein and how processed the food is.

This book's definition of 'healthy' means something that is not overly processed, has zero trans-fat, gives your body a benefit or energy when eaten and will not give you a diet related disease if eaten in moderation or often.

In summary: Myth vs. Reality

Myth: "Organic = Healthy."

Reality: Organic junk food is still junk food.

Myth: "Low-fat = Better."

Reality: Low-fat foods often replace fat with sugar.

Myth: "Sustainable = Nutritious."

Reality: Sustainability addresses environmental impact, not health.

🔍 **Food detectives shop smarter tip!**

How to spot "Health washing"

Ask these questions next time you shop:

Is it using words like sustainable, healthy, fresh and real?

Is the claim vague? ("Wholesome Goodness").

Does the nutrition label contradict the front-of-package claims? (e.g., "high-protein" bars with sugar as the first ingredient).

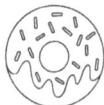

The issue with the word NATURAL

When someone hears the word 'natural', people assume green, nature, clean, pure, naked, free from "processedness". It is like how the word 'healthy' is used.

Many food companies and marketers love the word 'natural' because it is very ambiguous and it is not regulated. However, under any kind of food legislation, there is no legal definition of what qualifies as a 'natural food'. FSANZ (Food Standards Australia New Zealand), FDA (U.S.) and EFSA (Europe) have no official rules for what makes a food "natural." Hence why it's a big grey area that consumers are confused about, believing they are doing themselves a favour by eating 'natural foods' and food marketers can use this ambiguity to their advantage and can list 'natural' where they deem it fits their category positioning and branding.

Let's have a look at the dictionary meaning of food:

Natural: existing or derived from nature, not made or caused by humankind.

In terms of 'natural food', the public may believe that it is raw, unprocessed, organic, pure, wholesome or all the above.

However, some so-called 'natural foods' are just as processed as everything else, it really depends on what the ingredients are and how the ingredients are perceived by the consumer.

The word "natural" is one of the most powerful and misleading terms in food marketing. When consumers see it, they often picture fresh, unprocessed, chemical-free foods straight from nature. But "natural" has no legal definition in most countries, allowing companies to slap it on everything from highly processed snacks to soda. Let's look at some examples:

Companies can call foods "natural" even if they contain:

- Refined sugars ("natural cane sugar" is still sugar)

- Processed oils ("natural" fried chips are still fried)

- Artificial flavours (if derived from "natural sources")

Consumer Perception vs. Reality

5. The Marketing Tri Factor

What people think "natural" means:

- Unprocessed
- No artificial additives
- Farm-fresh, minimally altered

What it often means in practice:

At least one ingredient came from nature (even if heavily processed).

Example: "Natural" fruit snacks may contain 5% fruit juice and 95% sugar.

The "Processed but Natural" Trick

Many foods labelled "natural" undergo heavy processing:

"Natural" deli meats → Still contain nitrates and preservatives.

"Natural" peanut butter → Often has added hydrogenated oils.

"Natural" flavoured water → May include synthetic citric acid.

Examples of "natural" health washing: "Natural" is a marketing term, not a health guarantee. Just because something is labelled "natural" doesn't mean it's unprocessed, nutritious, or even safe in large amounts.

Food doesn't need a "natural" label.

For Foods Sake

Look out for the "natural" claims

Product	Claim	Reality
Natural cereal	Made with whole grains!	Contains refined flour + sugar as top ingredients
Natural soda	No artificial flavours!	Still contains sugar or artificial sweeteners.
All-natural "home-made" frozen dinner	No preservatives!	High in sodium, processed starches, and additives.
Natural candy	Real fruit extracts!	Little actual fruit content with refined sugar and food colouring

"Natural" is a marketing term, not a health guarantee. Just because something is labelled "natural" doesn't mean it's unprocessed, nutritious, or even safe in large amounts.

Food doesn't need a "natural" label.

🔍 Food detectives shop smarter tip!

How to avoid the "natural" trap

Ask yourself:
"What is the word NATURAL really distracting me from?"

Ignore front-label claims – Always check the ingredients list.

Look for certifications – If a product is truly minimally processed, it may have:

"100% Organic" (USDA/EU Organic logo)

"Non-GMO Verified" (this doesn't mean unprocessed)

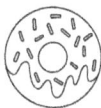

If you find that there are sugars, salts, sweeteners or flavour enhancers in it then it hardly qualifies as natural.

Why 'real', 'no nasties' are meaningless words

The word 'nasties' really means nothing, its marketing speak to scare you into thinking that the company's product is better and that their competitors have the so-called 'nasties'.

The word 'nasties' is a marketing term to scare consumers about the use of additives. Almost all processed food would have some use of additives, processing aid (a substance intentionally added during food processing to perform a specific technological function, like improving efficiency or quality. It does not perform a significant technological function in the final food product, or is used up, for example enzymes that are gone by the time the food is in final product form. These don't have to be declared in the ingredients list) or processed in a way that a consumer could not do without a manufacturing plant.

The term 'nasties' is a way to make it sound like certain ingredients that cannot be pronounced (they can be) are harmful. People have been conditioned to fear these "scary" sounding ingredients. Here's the thing, even natural ingredients, when broken down into their chemical components and using scientific names, will sound just as scary as the 'nasties'.

For example, if you break down the blueberry or banana right down to its chemical components, you will not want to eat it at all just based on how those chemical compounds sound like.

The word 'chemical' gets thrown around a lot from bloggers, influencers, nutritionists as if it's a dangerous corrosive substance that is bound to do harm to the human body. Chemicals are fundamental science, and marketers take advantage of the fact that these ingredients are 'scary' sounding and use it as a means to make a product seem healthier when it actually isn't.

There is a notion going around not to eat anything that your grandma doesn't recognise or ingredients that your grandma wouldn't recognise. This was a popular notion among the masses before the word 'nasties' became popular and the fear of ingredients that contain words such as 'acid' were deemed to be acceptable in mainstream society.

Now a lot of these ingredients have been rebranded into something that sounds less scary to the consumer. Instead of colouring, or natural colouring, there might be ingredients called 'natural black carrot colour' to denote that the colouring comes from black carrots in order to give the consumer a little bit of confidence that is where it comes from.

I will cover what the additives, 'chemicals', 'nasties' are for what they really are in the next chapter.

The word 'real' is also a misnomer where it is used to imply that all processed foods are not using 'real' ingredients. This implies that it is 'better' for you, and its ingredient list will still have an ingredient that is nowhere near the ingredient in its original or 'real' state. Any product that states it is 'natural' or 'real', should make you sceptical, and prompt you to read the actual ingredients list. If the product doesn't have any of the 'nasties', it still would have been processed to a degree that would make it debatable if it's still 'real'.

Food companies love using vague, feel-good words like "natural," "real," and "no nasties" to make their products seem healthier. But these terms are designed to manipulate, not inform. Here's why they're mostly meaningless, and how to see through the hype:

1. The fear-based marketing of "No Nasties"

What they want you to believe:

"Our product is pure; others are full of scary chemicals!"

"If you can't pronounce an ingredient, it must be bad for you!"

The Reality:

"Nasties" is not a scientific term; it's a marketing scare tactic.

All foods are made of chemicals (even water is H_2O).

Unpronounceable ≠ unsafe. Example:

"Ascorbic acid" = Vitamin C.

"Sodium chloride" = Table salt.

"Alpha-tocopherol" = Vitamin E.

The hypocrisy of "chemical fear"

If we broke down a banana into its chemical components, it would sound "scary" too:

Ethyl acetate (fruity ester)

Isoamyl acetate (part of banana flavour)

Polyphenol oxidase (enzyme that turns bananas brown)

Would you avoid bananas because of these names? Probably not, so why fear them in other foods?

How companies rebrand "scary" ingredients

Instead of:

"Citric acid" (a natural preservative from citrus)

They now say:

"Naturally derived from lemons!"

Instead of:

"Monosodium glutamate (MSG)" (a naturally occurring amino acid)

They now say:

"Natural Umami seasoning from tomatoes!"

This is the same ingredient, just repackaged to sound "cleaner."

2. The "real" food fallacy

What they claim:

"Our product is made with real ingredients!"

"No fake stuff!"

The Truth:

"Real" is an unregulated term. A "real fruit snack" might contain 5% fruit powder and 95% sugar.

Processing changes "real" ingredients. Example:

"Real cheese" on frozen pizza = heavily processed cheese product.

"Real honey" in cereal = mixed with syrups and additives.

The "Grandma Test" Myth

"Don't eat anything your grandma wouldn't recognise!"

Problem: Your grandma wouldn't recognise "xanthan gum," but it's just a fermented polysaccharide (complex sugar) used to thicken foods (like in salad dressings).

Many safe, modern ingredients sound unfamiliar but aren't harmful.

🔍 **Food detectives shop smarter tip!**

How to spot the marketing fearmongering?

Ask yourself:
"Is this just rebranded fearmongering?"

"No nasties" means nothing legally.

Learn basic food science – Not all additives are bad (e.g., pectin in jam is natural).

Chemicals aren't inherently bad (you're made of them too, we are all walking chemicals).

Processing isn't evil, it's about degree and purpose.
Judge food by its nutrition, not its packaging or marketing.

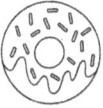

Stop being worried about the word CHEMICAL

The word chemical has been thrown about a lot in the nutrition, influencer and social media and it has been used in a way that makes anything that contains CHEMICALS into something that is toxic and negative. Chemical as a word has been weaponised to make consumers fear anything associated with the word nasties, which is a commonly used word by food marketing to make you think a food is healthier than it is.

Do these phrases sound familiar?

"These products have all kinds of chemicals that we don't know about, and they're loaded with nasties, e-numbers that nobody understands!"

"No nasties, No chemicals, only natural ingredients"

If you see any of these marketing words, it typically means marketers are disguising the food as something else or using "nasties" as a red herring. The reason why food marketers love using and exploiting chemophobia is because it triggers an evolutionary bias that fears the "unknown" or so-called "unnatural" substances and with the added fear of 'if it's hard to pronounce, it must be a risk' (Song & Schwarz, 2009). Consumers will often misinterpret chemical names as dangerous which creates a false dichotomy between "clean" and "processed" foods. These statements are classic examples of the 'chemical fallacy'. ALL substances are chemicals, including water (H_2O), oxygen (O_2) and vitamins. Also, many natural substances are in fact toxic such as arsenic and cyanide while additives and E-numbers mean they have gone through extensive testing before they can be used in any kind of food processing (Magnuson et al., 2013).

The reality is that all foods are in fact made entirely of chemicals.

So, the next time you see any marketing claim that says on the packaging "Free of nasties", "No chemicals", it should raise a red flag that this is poor food marketing and often means they are trying to distract you from something else.

How are serving sizes used in food marketing?

Serving sizes are dictated by the food manufacturer/producer, the serving size of a food is the recommended quantity that a consumer would 'typically' eat in one sitting.

However, this depends on several things:

- The type of product
- The size of the packaging
- The packaging type
- How it is being consumed

Serving sizes can make sense but sometimes they don't to the consumer. When working in the food industry, we dictate the serving size, and this is usually done alongside the marketing team.

The type of product will dictate the serving size whether it's a solid, to be cooked, ready to eat or to be eaten over different eating times.

For example, breakfast cereals. These would have a serving size of approximately 40g and if it's a 400g packet, that means there are 10 serves in that packet.

In the food industry, to get to the 40g, we would get an 'average' sized bowl. Some companies are more exact and precise when it comes to selecting what the 'average' sized bowl would look like. The 40g would have been selected mainly based on how 'full' looking it is in the bowl. However, no consumer would know what the 'average' bowl would look like, and an 'average' bowl would be subjective to each consumer hence why the true serving size is going to be different for everyone.

Shrinkflation: The art of distraction in food marketing

Shrinkflation, a covert strategy employed by food manufacturers, involves reducing the size or quantity of a product while maintaining its price. This tactic can be remarkably subtle, often going unnoticed by consumers. Food manufacturers deploy marketers who have mastered the art of selling you less for the same price, often without you noticing. Shrinkflation is often disguised by clever rebranding, flashy packaging, and marketing sleight of hand.

It is now becoming increasingly prevalent in a cost-of-living crisis where consumers are noticing that their processed foods are not the same size or weight.

Shrinkflation works because consumers are more sensitive to price hikes than subtle size reductions. Instead of raising prices (which would trigger backlash), companies:

- Reduce product size (e.g., 500g → 450g)
- Keep the price the same (or even increase it)
- Distract you with rebranding

Why does shrinkflation work and why do marketers love it? Marketers are aware that our brains prioritise visual cues over numbers. A "new look" tricks us into thinking we're getting something better. It's easy to assume packaging changes mean improvements, not downsizing.

Food marketers use packaging, rebrands and visual updates either in isolation or in combination to distract the consumer from the shrinkflation. Retailers don't mind this either as it doesn't affect their margins too much so long as they can keep their shelf configurations with little disruption. The reason why food companies do this is to ensure they can achieve margins and profitability. Remember they are also businesses that need to survive, and this is one of the ways they do this.

Sometimes a change in packaging, branding or front of pack claims is driven by competition, trends etc and food marketers also reduce the amount of product at the same time to disguise a change. Usually, the changes in reduction of food products are done incrementally over time and not in a sudden change in weight, for example 100g down to 95g won't be noticeable but 100g to 70g will be.

The psychology of packaging

Packaging plays a pivotal role in consumer perception. When a product is rebranded or its visuals are updated, it can create a sense of novelty and improvement. Consumers may be drawn to the fresh look and feel, associating it with better quality or enhanced value. This psychological trick can distract them from noticing the actual reduction in product quantity.

Colour and design

Bright, eye-catching colours and modern designs can captivate consumers. By focusing on the aesthetics, shoppers may overlook changes in package size.

Font and messaging

Using different fonts and messaging can alter the perceived value of the product. Phrases like "new and improved" can lead consumers to believe they are getting a better deal.

Updated claims

Showing new claims such as 'Gluten-free' whilst keeping the branding and packaging the same is a common way of reducing the amount of product.

Rebranding strategies

Rebranding is a powerful strategy that can mask shrinkflation. When a product undergoes a complete makeover, from its name to its logo, it can create an illusion of positive change. Consumers might be willing to pay the same price or even more for what appears to be a premium, updated version of the product, despite receiving less.

Name change: Altering the product name can refresh its identity and make it seem different, even though the core product remains the same.

Logo Redesign: A new logo can signal innovation and attract attention away from the reduced quantity.

Rebranding is often a risky exercise for food marketers as it can make or break consumer trust and goodwill, and if a product has been enjoyed by consumers, any changes can cause an uproar on social media and loss of sales.

Visual updates

Visual updates, including changes in packaging graphics, can serve as a distraction technique. By drawing the consumer's attention to the visual aspects, manufacturers can subtly reduce the product size without causing alarm.

Graphics and Imagery: High-resolution images and appealing graphics can elevate the perceived value.

Product Placement: Strategic placement of visual elements can emphasize certain aspects, diverting attention from the size.

Here are some of examples that food marketers use:

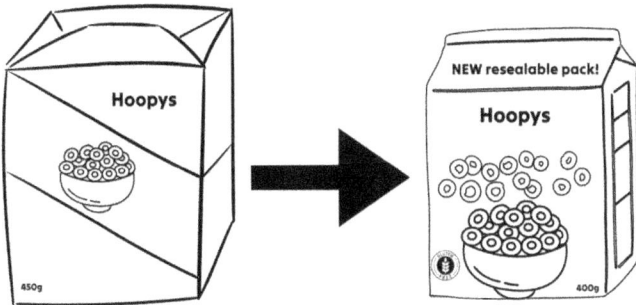

#1: The "New & Improved" Rebrand

Old packaging: "Classic Recipe!"

New packaging: "Now Even Better! And Gluten Free" (but 10% smaller and it was always gluten free now with just a bold claim on the front of the pack)

5. The Marketing Tri Factor

Example: A cereal box shrinks from 450g to 400g, but the bold new design makes it seem "premium" and a big claim stating the cereal is gluten-free even when it was always gluten-free to begin with.

#2: The "Sleek Makeover" Distraction

Before: A chunky, straightforward package.

After: A slim, "eco-friendly" redesign (with 15% less product).

Example: A chocolate bar goes from 100g to 85g, but the thinner wrapper makes it look "more elegant or sleek" or the chocolate bar itself has a different shape.

#3: The "Convenience" excuse

Claim: "New easy-pour spout!" or "Resealable pack!"

Reality: The bottle is now shorter and wider, holding less liquid.

Example: Juice bottles shrink from 1L to 900mL, but the new shape makes it harder to compare.

Examples of shrinkflation

Product	Old size	New size	Claim tactic used
Chips	200g bag	180g bag	New crunchier texture!
Ice Cream	1L tub	800ml tub	Creamier recipe!
Instant coffee	500g jar	450g jar	Bolder flavour
Milk chocolate	250g	200g	Made with real milk

Food companies have been getting away with this as most shoppers don't weigh or measure products. Typically, consumers would trust brands and labels without questioning them and supermarkets rarely flag size reductions as it's not in the best interest to do so either.

Shrinkflation is a deceptive food marketing practice of hiding price increases that relies heavily on the power of rebranding, visual updates, and new packaging. These marketing strategies can effectively distract consumers, making it difficult for them to notice that they are getting less for their money. By staying alert to packaging tricks, rebranding, and shrinking sizes, you can avoid paying more for less.

The next time you see a "new look", "new claim", "new packaging" of a food product, look out for shrinkflation!

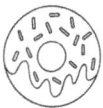

🔍 **Food detectives shop smarter tip!**

How to spot shrinkflation

Ask yourself:
"What's really changed here?"

Read product labels and compare weights and sizes.

Check unit pricing – Look for price per 100g/mL (not just total cost).

Compare old vs. new packaging – Hold them side by side if possible.

Ignore "new look" claims – Focus on weight and size, not marketing buzzwords.

Complain when you see it – Companies backtrack when consumers notice (e.g., Toblerone's 2016 shrinkflation backlash)

How food marketing disguises 'flavoured' food and what to look out for

If a food product is flavoured, it must state so. There are many ultra processed foods that are flavoured which are typically in the foods that are the 'guilty pleasures' that don't have any of the ingredient that the flavour is naming on the front of the packet.

For example, you would have drinks that are blueberry flavoured. However, this means that there is no blueberry ingredient in those drinks.

The word flavour is usually in smaller font. There are some products that will also state that they use natural flavours.

I will go over the types of flavour classifications in a different chapter.

The Marketing Tri factor check

The next time you walk down the supermarket aisle, remember this:

Food marketing isn't designed to help you make better choices; it's designed to sell more to you. They don't want to feel responsible for your health and they shouldn't be. Their job is to ensure that they meet their own Key Performance Indicators (KPIs) such as sales, market share, and profit margins and this is often prioritised over consumer well-being.

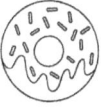

🔍 **Marketing Tri Factor check**

Ask yourself from a consumers perspective (you):

"Who am I as a consumer?"

"What am I trying to achieve in my lifestyle with these products?"

"Am I purchasing this product based on impulse or nostalgia?"

"If I can make this at home, would it still appeal to me?"

"Does this copy resonate with me or is it just buzz words?"

"What claims are on here?"

"What claims are NOT on here?"

"How many times does the marketing on this pack use words such as natural, real, no nasties?"

"Am I buying this for the taste or for a specific claim?"

Conclusion: The Marketing Tri Factor

During my undergrad in food technology, I helped volunteer in the national ice cream awards. This involved preparing samples and of course, trying those samples myself. This was a highlight of my studies and being able to eat all the ice cream from all over the country was a great way to try all the different flavours at the time like chocolate raspberry ganache, salted caramel miso, it was great! As I'm preparing the samples, the organiser tells me to stop. They looked at the packaging and told me that one of the entries was disqualified. I ask them why.

They show me the packaging and tell me that it is not ice cream. I look closely and sure enough the packaging says it's a 'frozen dessert'. Sure enough, I didn't realise at the time there was an actual difference between ice cream and frozen dessert. In New Zealand, they take their ice cream very seriously. Now from the initial appearance, it looks like ice cream from the packaging. It was intentionally marketed this way.

5. The Marketing Tri Factor

Frozen dessert often gets away with looking like ice cream when it's really not. The difference between ice cream and frozen dessert is the milk fat content and frozen dessert can be made with vegetable oils. Frozen desserts typically have more air and stabilisers which make it cheaper to produce. The organiser who was also a food technologist showed me how the marketing was used to make you think something that isn't true. They were using the words of flavours in big colourful font like "Simply Vanilla" and with the frozen dessert words hidden on the bottom left corner and just legible enough to be legal. Ever since then, I have always ignored what the marketing says and look out for the legal definition of a product.

Now that we understand how emotional tugs, nostalgia, claims, romance copy and consumer lifestyles have been weaponised against the consumer, we are now seeing food marketing for what it is. A way to make you consume more and become a repeat customer.

It's best to know where you stand in your lifestyle, values, habits so that you're not swayed or fooled by the marketing gimmicks and tricks that have been shown to you here.

Also of course if you feel like a trip down memory lane, there is no harm in doing so. Every processed and ultra processed food probably has been a part of your childhood to some extent and going back for a little trip is not harmful, but it can do some damage when the nostalgia trips become a part of your daily habit.

If nothing else, the claims on the pack are what I want everyone in this book to pay close attention to. If a product is claiming something on the front of the pack, think also what they're NOT claiming and ALWAYS look at the ingredients list and the nutritional panel.

Remember that the marketing is part of the experience but don't let it fool you into buying something that you're not looking for.

6. The Consumption Tri Factor

What drives us to purchase and consume one food product over another? In this chapter, we will deep dive into the Consumption Tri Factor which is all about the taste, price and convenience of food products. These three things are the main factors on what makes us purchase food whether consciously or unconsciously.

We've explored how the irresistible Tri Factor is used to get you hooked and consume to give you a consistent sensory experience every time, combined with the Marketing Tri Factor that makes you blissfully unaware of the branding deception that happens. Both these tri factors are what ultimately lead to the Consumption Tri Factor. With the ongoing cost-of-living crisis, the price and affordability of food is a big factor for many households whether a food product is purchased or not. We'll reverse engineer the tactics and get into a deep dive of the science of flavours, decoding the nutritional information panel and what the food industry is doing to improve and where it's still falling short.

The Consumption Tri Factor are the three things that consumers focus on when they purchase food. This chapter will reverse engineer what the food companies do to get you to purchase a product, combined with the Marketing Tri Factor we've already covered.

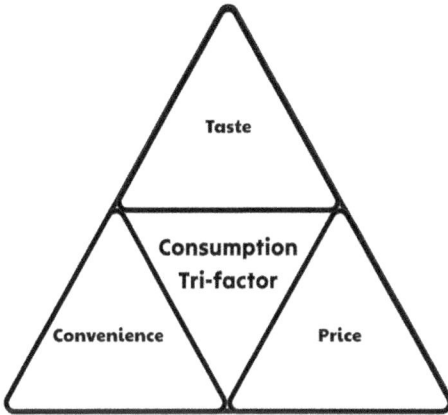

Convenience: More than just the packaging

Unless you're buying fresh fruits and vegetables without packaging, almost all processed foods will have some form of packaging which gives us consumers the convenience of taking food home and being able to store it. Packaging in general is an important part of the Consumption Tri Factor which determines the convenience and price of a product. In this section, we'll cover the following:

- The different types of packaging and their functions
- How marketing shapes packaging design
- Why packaging goes beyond mere food safety
- The psychology behind supermarket product placement

Different types of packaging

Packaging is the one of the first interactions you will have with a food product (with the exception of those promotional people giving away free samples of promoted food products at the supermarket). Its form, appearance, texture, weight and materials are all part of the experience when you're purchasing a food product. Even the sound of the crinkling of a chip bag. The experience of grabbing that packaging and putting it into your shopping trolley, carrying it to your car, and then storing it in your fridge and how you dispose of it (or hopefully recycle it) are all part of the packaging experience.

At its core, the main functions of packaging are:

- Protection: By keeping food safe from contamination, moisture, and spoilage.
- Portability: Ensuring food can be transported efficiently from factory to shelf.
- Persuasion: Making the product marketable and visually appealing to stand out in a crowded market.

Food safety is the paramount function, and packaging is a key component of making food safe to eat. When product development and packaging technologists are creating new products, packaging is one of the things they must consider for both the consumer and the manufacturing site. Consumer perception of packaging materials plays into how it can be marketed. At the same time, it must be able to keep food safe, transportable and easily stored.

These are materials that are used and are all part of keeping food safe. They usually have different levels explained below:

Primary packaging

This is the packaging that is in direct contact with the food, it is important that this is either sealed or airtight and keeps the food secure. The primary packaging ensures that food isn't going to be contaminated by any external sources such as microbial, chemical or sunlight (Robertson, 2016).

Secondary packaging

This is the packaging that keeps the primary packaging and the product itself, transportable and presentable. Think of the cardboard box that cereals have. This is the packaging that makes it easy for consumers to purchase and store the product. Not all foods have secondary packaging, and it is only needed if the primary packaging isn't sufficient to make the item transportable. If secondary packaging is required, then it will be designed to catch your eye and make storage easy.

Tertiary packaging

Tertiary packaging usually is the large packaging that makes food products transportable between stores and distribution centres. These are usually cardboard boxes or RSCs (Regular Slotted Carton), shipping boxes, pallets and bulk containers where typically the consumer doesn't see these at all (Marsh & Bugusu, 2007).

Marketing designs, and the fluffy romance copy on the packaging

If you remove all the pretty colours, logos, text, images from food packaging, it will look bland and unappealing, and one would argue that this is exactly what should happen to make food more transparent. However, as consumers, we do look for brands that appeal to us and we think represent good quality products.

Without making food products appealing before we can get to eat them, the marketing, artwork and colours must give us a reason to purchase it.

Before any marketing is applied there is some crucial legal information that must be on the packaging, these are not optional and must be on the pack and where the consumer can read it. If the following is not on the pack, then it is liable to be recalled from the distributor:

Weight

Consumers need to know how much they are buying. These are usually in metric units in Europe, Australia, New Zealand, Japan, Southeast Asia etc.

There are different types of weight declarations:

Net weight

Net weight is the most used weight declaration of food where it is the weight of the food itself and not including the packaging. The easiest way to know the net weight is to take a bowl and scale and put in how much food product is from the pack. Typically, food producers will put in slightly more than the net weight to ensure they are compliant with what they are declaring.

Gross weight

Gross weight is the weight of the food including the food itself and the packaging. This is not commonly used however some food producers show both the gross and net weight of a product.

Average weight (also seen with the 'e' symbol next to the number)

The average weight for a product is for products where the food producer cannot guarantee the actual weight of the product. This is applied to products where there is a natural variation in the type of the weight, these products include chicken pieces, whole chicken etc.

Ingredients list

The ingredients list is an important piece of information for consumers. In New Zealand and Australia, ingredients are listed in descending order, by quantity. By law, all the ingredients in the food product must be listed.

Country of origin

Every food product must declare where it is made, produced or packaged. It is not legal to sell products without this. In Australia, the country of origin is more detailed where it lists out the amount of Australian ingredients. Each country has its own requirements and can differ.

As a consumer who wants to support local products, always look out for where the product is made. It will usually be listed on the back of the packaging.

Be careful with products that pretend to be locally made by using local or heritage images but are actually made and/or packaged somewhere else.

Product description

A product description is the basic descriptor for the product. Instead of Susan's delicious chocolate chip cookie. Its product description would be chocolate chip cookie.

Packaging information

Some countries also show the type of packaging so that consumers can make decisions on how to dispose or recycle their packaging properly. Some countries will state whether the packaging is recyclable or if it needs to be thrown in the bin. Below is an example of what they could look like:

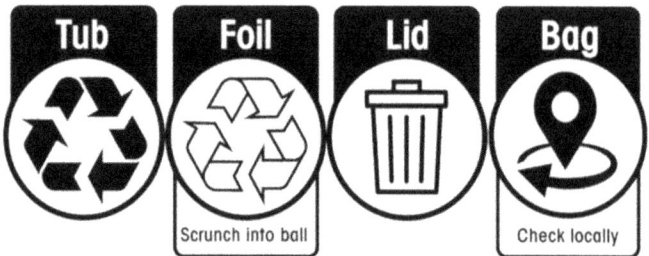

Source: Australian Recycling Label

Business address and information

Every food product must show some form of contact information so a consumer can reach out and make an inquiry. Typically, this is an address, company name and phone number.

For Foods Sake

Nutrition information

This is either called Nutritional Information or Nutritional Facts in North America and Canada. This important piece of information tells you the amount of energy and macronutrients (protein, carbohydrates and fats) in the food product. There are typically two columns they will be displayed which is the quantity per serve and the quantity per 100g.

Barcode (only small packs are exempt from this)

Barcodes on food packaging primarily serve to facilitate efficient inventory management, streamline checkout processes, and enhance traceability and food safety within the food supply chain. Many supermarkets, retailers and suppliers required a GS1 (Global Standards 1) barcode. GS1 allows food products to have more detailed information such as expiry dates, batch numbers, variants etc.

Allergen information

Every food product must declare the allergens on the packaging. If allergens are present and not declared, it could lead to a criminal charge and lawsuits against the food manufacturer. The allergen information would typically show the ingredients which are allergens in BOLD to make it obvious. These would say something like CONTAINS: MILK, PEANUTS. Or May Contain: WHEAT.

A "may contain" statement means that the product was made on a premises or with a process that may contain traces of those allergens. All food businesses must adhere to using PEAL (Plain English Allergen Labelling).

Best before/Use by date

Every food product has either a best before or use by date. In Australia and New Zealand, the best before date is an indication of the quality of the product that is best consumed before that date however it doesn't mean it can't be consumed past that date.

While the use by date is an indication of food safety where the food must be consumed before that date, these are usually for fresh or refrigerated products.

If a product looks off or something doesn't smell or taste right, you should dispose of it regardless of the best before or use by date.

Storage conditions

The storage conditions must also be shown on the packaging and is usually on the back. Storage conditions usually tell the consumer the best way to store the food when it has been opened or taken out of the packaging. Usually they would say something like 'store at room temperature' or 'keep refrigerated'.

Beyond these basics listed, packaging is a powerful storytelling tool. A luxury chocolate brand might use foil stamping and matte finishes to convey premium quality, while a budget snack might rely on bright colours and bold claims ("Now with 20% more!").

How marketing influences packaging

When it comes to how consumers view packaging, we'll focus on the primary and secondary packaging and how it is used to get you as a consumer to purchase processed food.

The primary and sometimes the secondary packaging is often changed to make it appealing to a consumer. This can be to the type of packaging that affects how it appears on the shelf. Because consumers have a very low attention span in the supermarket, it must stand out. Also, it must meet the supermarket requirements of being able to take up certain shelf space otherwise it will not be stocked. For packaging specialists, these are the things to consider on top of the materials which are now becoming more recyclable or at least made from recyclable materials.

At the time of writing this book, the supermarkets have started to mandate that the food packaging must be recyclable and/or be made from recyclable materials. However, this is a challenge when some materials (like multi-layer films) remain difficult to recycle, and alternatives can be prohibitively expensive (Verghese et al., 2015).

Additionally, recycling capabilities vary by region and what's recyclable in one city may end up in a landfill elsewhere.

Supermarket psychology: The positioning of products in supermarkets

When you walk into a supermarket, every product's placement from the entrance to the checkout aisle is meticulously planned to maximise sales. Food manufacturers and retailers use a combination of psychology, marketing, and data analytics to influence what you buy. Understanding these tactics can help you make more informed choices rather than falling prey to strategic product positioning.

1. The power of eye-level placement

Supermarkets know that consumers are more likely to buy products placed at eye level. This is why premium brands and higher-margin items are typically stocked where your gaze naturally falls. This is typically a height between 140cm to 190cm. Meanwhile, store-brand or healthier alternatives may be placed on higher or lower shelves, forcing you to actively search for them (Wansink, 2016).

2. Kid placement and impulse buys

Children's products (like sugary cereals) are often placed on lower shelves to be at a child's eye level, increasing "pester power" making it easier for little hands to grab and harder for parents to say no. For example, kids' yoghurt is always placed on the bottom aisle in the yoghurt section, and it is likely to have characters that kids love or cartoon animals to appeal to children with products that are not always great for children.

Impulse buys (candy, snacks, and cold carbonated beverages) are strategically positioned near checkout lanes where shoppers are more likely to grab them while waiting.

3. End of the line displays

End of line displays or the aisles closest to the cash registers/checkouts and are some of the most valuable spaces in a supermarket. These spots are often reserved for:

- Promotional items (discounted or seasonal products)
- New product launches (to attract attention)
- High margin processed foods (chips, sodas, frozen meals)

Retailers charge manufacturers hefty fees for these premium placements, meaning the products you see here are not necessarily the best choices, just the most profitable for the store. Note as well that a promoted product is not always the best value product.

4. The "Golden Zone" and the supermarket layout

Supermarkets are designed to guide you through a specific path:

Fresh produce is usually placed near the entrance to create a perception of freshness and health. Almost all the fresh produce like vegetables, fruits, meats, and perishables are all on the edge of the supermarket. Refrigerated and frozen foods are situated at the back as it's easier to maintain from a supermarket perspective.

Staple items (milk, eggs, bread) are often at the back of the store, forcing you to walk past other tempting products which are usually ultra processed foods.

6. The Consumption Tri Factor

Processed and snack foods dominate the centre aisles, where shoppers spend the most time browsing.

This layout ensures maximum exposure to high-profit items before you reach your essentials.

5. How supermarkets and food companies negotiate placement

Supermarkets don't just randomly assign shelf space; there's a financial and psychological game behind it.

Slotting fees: Food manufacturers pay supermarkets for prime shelf positions. Big brands with deep pockets can afford the best spots, while smaller, healthier brands may be pushed to less visible areas.

Planograms: These are detailed maps of where each product should go, often influenced by sales data and manufacturer agreements rather than consumer health.

Private-label products: Many supermarkets prioritise their own store-brand items (which have higher profit margins) over or next to name brands, placing them in more prominent locations.

Q Food detectives shop smarter tip!

Now that you know how supermarkets manipulate product placement, here's how to take back control:

Look beyond eye level: Healthier or budget-friendly options if they exist are often above or below eye level so be sure to scan the shelves in all directions.

Stick to a list: Avoid impulse buys triggered by strategic displays and clever placement.

Shop the perimeter first: Fresh produce, dairy, and meats are usually along the edges, while processed foods dominate the centre aisles.

By understanding these tactics, you can navigate the supermarket with a critical eye and make choices that align with your health and budget, rather than the store's bottom line.

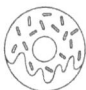

Price: Paying for convenience and quality

Price and convenience are the parts of this tri factor that are very intertwined with quality, perception (marketing budgets) and positioning in the supermarket. The price of any food product is the negotiation between perceived quality, convenience and marketing influence. When you're buying a food product, it's not just the ingredients that you're paying for. You're paying for the labour, packaging, branding and the psychological position of where it sits in the supermarket.

So, what really goes into that price and how to spot when you're paying for actual value versus clever marketing tactics?

Every food product's cost is shaped by multiple factors, some obvious, some hidden:

Branding & marketing: A well-known brand can charge more simply because consumers trust it, even if the ingredients are nearly identical to a cheaper alternative (Aaker, 1996).

Ingredients: Higher-quality (or perceived higher-quality) ingredients cost more. Organic, free-range, or imported components drive prices up, but don't always guarantee better taste or nutrition.

Processing & labour: Handmade, small-batch, or artisanal products (like gourmet granola or craft ice cream) cost more because of time-intensive production.

6. The Consumption Tri Factor

Format & convenience: Pre-shredded cheese, single-serve yoghurt pouches, or pre-cut vegetables save you time, but you pay extra for that convenience.

Packaging: Fancy looking jars, resealable bags, or portion-controlled packs add to the cost.

Supply chain: Where it's made, stored (ambient, chilled, or frozen), and transported affects the price. Imported goods often cost more due to tariffs and logistics.

Supermarket markup & positioning: Stores take a cut, and premium shelf placement (eye-level, endcaps) isn't free, brands pay for those spots (Wansink, 2016).

Below is a checklist of food pricing and why you pay more for perception. Use these the next time you're in the supermarket shopping.

1. The "loss leader" trap

Typically, the price of the food product is determined by the branding/marketing, this influences the position in the supermarket shelves. If a product can be sold in higher volumes even at a lower price point, then businesses would allow that, and this is called a loss leader where they have a product that takes the brunt of the losses, but the profit is made up with other products (Hui et al., 2013).

This is why rotisserie chickens are sold on the cheap, it's a classic supermarket loss leader product sold at a loss to lure you in, hoping you'll buy higher-margin items alongside them, such as a salad and bread rolls.

2. The convenience premium

The format of a product is important to determine how much it will cost, typically this will be its packaging or changing the product's form to be more convenient for the customer.

An example of this is shredded cheese. This may seem like an overly simple example however the product of shredded cheese is exactly the type of convenience that many families are looking for. Instead of shredding cheese yourself which can be a cumbersome task for some, by paying slightly more, this becomes a far easier option when preparing meals at home. As a caveat, for shredded cheese to last longer, it requires anti-caking agents, so it doesn't stick together and preservatives, so it doesn't become mouldy.

Another example is yoghurt and its different packaging formats. The yoghurt inside a 1L tub is the same if it is put in a 250ml tub or a 200ml pouch or at least let's assume this is true in this example. The difference between these is the fact that a 250ml tub is more convenient in a lunch box. However, a 200ml pouch is even more convenient than a 250ml tub as you don't need a spoon to consume it. What happens is that because of the convenience, you as the consumer will be charged at a higher rate per kilo of yoghurt. Either option works for your lifestyle, and it depends on your views on reducing packaging, waste, preparation etc.

3. The "Health halo" Effect

Words like *organic*, *artisanal*, or *craft* make us assume a product is better, even if it's not. A study found consumers willingly paid **up to 23% more** for foods labelled "organic," regardless of actual quality (Lee et al., 2013). If a product is perceived to have better quality ingredients, typically the food manufacturer must justify why on the pack, then they can charge a higher premium. However just because something is perceived to have better quality ingredients doesn't mean it's going to be a superior product.

Some products have more expensive and labour-intensive processing. Such products can include gourmet granola or muesli, meat pies or handmade ice cream. There are products where the processing is still novel or new, requires more ingredients than other products in its range such as gourmet yoghurt that don't have any thickeners and are using premium cultures.

4. The novelty tax

New flavours or formats (like kombucha in a can vs. a bottle) often debut at higher prices. If they sell well, they might get cheaper, if not, they disappear. Some food companies will be clever in how they release certain products where they will release new flavours only in the larger or smaller pack sizes to gauge whether there is a demand for that product and if it will be successful.

How supermarkets play the pricing game

- **Eye-Level = High Profit** – Premium brands pay for prime shelf space. Store-brand alternatives (often just as good) are usually on the bottom shelf.
- **Anchor pricing** – A $10 "gourmet" sauce next to a $6 one makes the $6 option seem like a steal, even if it's normally $5.
- **Shrinkflation** – As mentioned previously in the Marketing Tri Factor, your favourite snack stays the same price but gets smaller (e.g., chocolate bars shrinking from 100g to 80g).

The price isn't just about the food; it's also about choices. Every time you buy groceries; you're voting with your wallet. Understanding why things cost what they do helps you decide:

- *Is this convenience worth it?*
- *Is this "premium" product actually better?*

Armed with this knowledge, you can outsmart pricing tricks and make choices that align with your budget, your values and make your dollar work smarter.

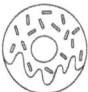

Q **Food detectives shop smarter tip!**

How to navigate supermarketing pricing:

Compare unit prices – Check the price per 100g/kg (usually in small print) to see which size or brand is truly cheaper.

Ask: "Am I paying for convenience or quality?" – Pre-cut veggies save time, but whole ones save money.

Beware of "premium" labels – Does "small-batch" or "handcrafted" actually mean better, or just pricier?

Try store brands – Many are made in the same factories as name brands, just without the fancy packaging.

Taste

Flavours

The world of food comprises the infinite possibility of flavours. Aside from the Irresistible Tri Factor, flavours give all food the extra dimension that makes eating give us an experience that none of the other senses can give.

In this chapter, we'll dive into the world of flavours, what they are, how they influence human taste, how they are produced, how flavours have been used in the industry, how marketing uses flavours to their advantage.

What is a flavour?

The definition of a flavour is the distinctive taste of that food or beverage.

Flavour is a combination of taste and aroma or smell.

Flavours come in many different forms. All foods have a flavour profile from mother nature, and there are many variations of flavours that come from different regions, cultures, climates and animal or plant species.

Flavour is also affected by processing, temperature, texture, packaging, chemical composition and the form it comes in.

Without flavour, the world would be boring. Flavour profiles of everyday foods, dishes and drinks are what makes our lives interesting. If everything were to taste the same, then we'd just be eating the same thing every day without complaint. But we are not such animals, flavour is multidimensional. It brings worlds together that collide beautifully.

Flavour is something that the food industry has much to be proud of albeit with a lot of science and creativity.

There is a product called Soylent which was made so that it would give you all your nutrients in a convenient drink. There was only one type of flavour, and the purpose of that drink was to replace meals thinking it would reduce waste, and overcome decision making fatigue.

The problem? People got sick of consuming the same thing every day. Even the owner of Soylent realised that they needed new flavours and variety in their diets to maintain their satiety and sanity. Humans crave variety, texture, and excitement in their food, it is in our DNA for survival. Our ancestors relied on taste and smell to avoid poison (bitter = danger) and seek nutrients (sweet = energy).

Taste is one of our primary senses and this allows us to experience flavour. There are 5 main different types of tastes (it's still debatable among the scientific community if it's just 5):

Sweet - from sugar, ripe fruit, honey

Salty - from salt, olives, cured meats

Sour - from lemon juice, vinegar, tangy yoghurt

Bitter - from black coffee, dark chocolate

Umami/Savoury - from MSG, mushrooms, soy sauce

Our tongue is our primary organ for taste and when you're younger it is easily influenced by the food that we eat. Some people are blessed with more tastebuds than others, these people are called supertasters. Our tastebuds take in the flavours of our food or drinks and tell the brain whether we should continue chewing or not.

Smell allows us to pick up the scents or aroma of a food that over years of evolution, gave us some indication if something was edible or not. Without aroma, you won't get much flavour out of anything.

Try this:

Pinch your nose and put some vanilla ice cream in your mouth and don't swallow. Notice that it doesn't taste as much vanilla as before, it will most likely taste bland. Release your nose, and now you can really get the vanilla flavours to come through. This is because 80% of flavour comes from smell (Spence, 2015).

How are flavours made

Flavours are made by a different variety of methods which are both a science and an art.

Natural flavours must be derived from plants, animals, or microbiological sources (FSANZ, 2023). Below is a short summary of the different processes which vary by ingredient and the type of flavour:

1. Distillation (For herbs, spices, citrus)

Steam distillation – Boiling plant material (e.g., peppermint leaves) to capture aromatic oils.

Cold pressing – Citrus peels are mechanically squeezed to extract oils (think: lemon zest in a bottle).

2. Fermentation (For umami, cheese, wine notes)

Microbes break down compounds into flavour-rich molecules:

Soy sauce – Fermented soybeans create savoury depth.

Vanilla – Cured orchid pods develop vanillin over months.

3. Enzymatic reactions (For buttery, meaty notes)

Enzymes in aged cheese or slow-roasted meat unlock rich, complex flavours.

4. Solvent extraction (For delicate flavours like rose)

Alcohol or CO_2 pulls flavours from fragile sources (e.g., saffron, vanilla beans).

"Natural" doesn't always mean "straight from the farm." A "natural strawberry flavour" might start with real fruit but undergo heavy processing to concentrate it. These processes are usually more expensive due to the sourcing of the original ingredient and processes. Natural flavours don't last as long as artificial flavours due to their high volatility.

Artificial flavours

Artificial flavours are chemically identical to natural ones but made by chemical synthesis. The process:

1. Gas chromatography-mass spectrometry (GC-MS)

Scientists "taste-test" a food (e.g., a ripe peach) using GC-MS machines that identify key compounds (e.g., gamma-decalactone = peachy sweetness) and break them down into their flavour molecules.

2. Lab replication

Chemists can recreate those molecules from petroleum byproducts or wood pulp (yes, really).

Example: Vanillin (the main flavour in vanilla) is often made from lignin, a paper industry waste product as natural vanilla is more expensive.

3. Blending

Single molecules rarely mimic a full flavour, so labs mix dozens (e.g., 50+ compounds for "tropical punch").

The Grey Area: "Nature-Identical" Flavours

Some flavours are synthetic copies of natural molecules but still labelled "natural" if chemically identical. For example:

"Natural" vanillin from fermented corn sugar (not vanilla orchids).

"Natural" almond flavour (benzaldehyde) from apricot pits.

In Australia, these can be called "natural" if the molecule exists in nature, even if it was made in a vat (FSANZ, 2023). As a consumer, you won't be able to know if a flavour is natural or nature identical as this is part of the food companies' intellectual property.

How are flavours used by marketers and food technologists?

Flavourings make certain taste profiles more accessible without the use of fresh ingredients. Using the actual ingredients for a flavour or to achieve a specific taste profile can be prohibitively expensive.

Some taste profiles are achieved with a variety of additives ranging from flavours, flavour enhancers and/ or sweeteners.

The best example of this are flavoured foods versus products with the actual ingredients.

Flavoured foods are disguised amongst the array of other products. Typically, these are cheaper than your other products because they don't contain the ingredient of the flavour they are showing on the front of the packet.

For example:

Maple and blueberry flavoured muesli bars.

6. The Consumption Tri Factor

Reading this it could imply that some blueberries or maple syrup are in it however with the way this is worded, it doesn't have to be.

If the word 'flavoured' or 'flavour' is on the front of the pack after the ingredient, it means that the manufacturer does NOT have to put in any ingredients but can put in flavour instead.

If it said "maple flavoured muesli bars with blueberries" then it means that it is maple flavoured with actual blueberries (in the case of a muesli bar, it would most likely be dried blueberries).

Sometimes the word 'flavour' would be in smaller text so the consumer can't readily see it. Food companies and marketing often hide the word in tiny text while highlighting images of fruit or the ingredient to trick your brain into thinking they are in it.

So, if there is strawberry yoghurt vs strawberry-flavoured yoghurt, the latter doesn't need to contain strawberries and most likely won't have any real strawberries in it.

This is very common in drinks and beverages where there are beverages, juices and drinks which all seem to blend in together.

Juice and fruit drinks are not the same.

Juice that is sold in the supermarket contains actual fruit or vegetable juice. The content of the juice will be dependent on what is put on the front of the packaging.

Juice can be either from concentrate, reconstituted, or fresh. Sometimes it is a combination of these processing methods where the juice is procured. Even if juice does not have any sugar added, it is still high in natural sugars.

Fruit drinks on the other hand typically contain less than 25% juice. Fruit drinks should really be called 'fruit flavoured' drinks. Because they typically have far more water and sugars than actual fruit juice. These would usually have obvious marketing that highlights the picture of the fruit and the words 'fruit drink' would be placed in very small font.

The best way to find out if a product is a fruit drink is to see if the word flavour and fruit drink is on the pack and check the ingredients list. If water is the first ingredient listed, it is more than likely to be a fruit drink.

You will see this very commonly with potato crisps as well. In potato crisps, flavourings are used to achieve the taste of what is being declared.

A very common flavour of crisps is BBQ-flavoured crisps, which uses a combination of flavours, salts, spices to achieve the taste.

Cheese-flavoured crisps usually have some form of cheese but it's not actual cheese, it would be a cheese flavour and sometimes a combination of cheese powder.

What is the deal with artificial flavours? Are they really that bad for you?

Many products on the supermarket shelves boast claims of no artificial flavours, colours or sweeteners.

Why is there so much hate for artificial flavours, and colours in particular?

Have we actually questioned why these are so hated by consumers? The artificial flavours, colours and sweeteners were deemed the original 'nasties'.

There was a study back in the 1990's where they gave children solutions of artificial flavours and colours and it was discovered that those children would go hyper with lots of energy.

When this study was released, the media took it and ran with it to make it sound like those artificial sweeteners and colours would make children hyperactive or even getting ADHD. When parents found out, they didn't want any artificial flavours or colours in their food which prompted the early precursor to those artificial flavours and colours to be seen as 'chemicals'.

However, if you read the paper, it was found that the solutions that contained the artificial colours and flavours were made with sugar solutions. So of course, those children were going to be jumping up and down (NIH, 2019). This study was rebuked, and it was not done in a scientific manner. However, the way it was reported in the media influenced how processed food is seen by the general public to this day and plays a part in how food is marketed.

Artificial colours, flavours and sweeteners are still in processed food. They are usually hidden in plain sight, so you wouldn't notice it. This is what the marketers do:

Instead of declaring what is artificial, they will highlight what ISN'T artificial. There are many products that still use artificial flavours or colours so instead the claims could be shown to see 'No artificial sweeteners' OR a positive claim like "Made with 25% orange juice!"

From a food technologists' perspective, the use of artificial additives like colours, flavours and sweeteners are all dependent on the type of product that needs to be made. Artificial flavours are often identical to natural ones at a molecular level (just cheaper and more stable). If an artificial flavour, colour or sweetener can be used, it makes our job a lot easier.

There are several reasons for this:

- Artificial additives are usually cheaper, real vanilla is 3000% more expensive than synthetic vanillin.

- They last longer and are more consistent than their natural counterparts which degrade faster.

- They are more resilient and able to withstand processing such as heat treatment, baking, frying, pasteurisation.

- They are less volatile, and you need to use less of it to achieve the same function as their natural counterparts.

Many products will have artificial additives, but you won't even notice it because generally speaking, if it tastes good, you won't taste the difference.

Flavours are far more powerful than consumers realise. They shape history, culture, and commerce. Understanding how they work, and how they're used to influence us, helps you eat smarter, shop wiser, and savour better. Flavours affect your purchasing decisions as well, if there is a flavour available for your product, the more likely you will buy it. Food technologists and marketers have used both actual flavours and the word flavour to get it associated with a food product you would have a positive affinity with which makes you susceptible to buying something you would try and or don't need.

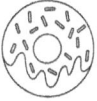

Unprocessed Imposters: What to look out for

There are many products on the supermarket shelves that give consumers the perception that they're not ultra processed and that they're healthy. In reality, they are no better than eating something that is heavily processed. Here are some imposters to look out for:

Dried fruit

Dried fruit is processed but the majority of the time still has its food matrix intact. It is typically accompanied with sugar and preservatives (usually in the form of sulphites). Look out for dried fruit that doesn't have preservatives or sugar, the caveat is that they don't last as long and are usually more expensive. Instead try opting for no sugar added dried fruit like Medjool dates or try making your own with a dehydrator.

Orange juice

Orange juice is very processed, and it has a variety of different forms. Even the cold pressed version will have high natural sugar content and will often lack fibre. Some orange juices can contain as much sugar as some sodas, so have a look at the nutritional label.

Plant-based milks

Almond, Oat and Soy milks have become very popular however the quantities of those ingredients in those milks are typically no more than 2%, and they usually contain emulsifiers, thickeners (like carrageenan), added sugars, and synthetic vitamins. These would usually have added calcium as there is legislation that those kinds of products have added calcium in them. It is best to purchase the plant-based milks with no added sugars and minimal thickeners.

Oat & Granola/Muesli Bars

These convenient snack bars are often loaded with added sugars, oils, and preservatives. Even "organic" or "natural" versions can be highly processed with refined sweeteners like brown rice syrup or maltodextrin. They often leverage oats as the healthy hero ingredient, and they are accompanied with marketing claims like "granola bar for energy".

Muesli and Granola

Mueslis are one of those products that seem very unprocessed however they contain many ingredients that you don't need. Because they contain ingredients that you would recognise, it's easy to assume they're unprocessed or healthy, however they would have oils, sugars, cereals like rice puffs to make it cheaper.

🍳 **Bonus Recipe!**

Make your own muesli - It is easy to make your own and it's far cheaper:

Ingredients:
Rolled Oats
Honey/Maple Syrup
Little bit of olive oil
Sunflower seeds
Whole or sliced Almonds
Coconut flakes (optional)

Put all of these in a mixing bowl and place on top of a baking sheet on a baking tray and lay it out flat. Bake for approximately 15 minutes at 160 degrees Celsius. Let it cool and break into pieces that are slightly joined together.

Cereals

There's no such thing as a 'healthy' cereal. These are some of the most highly processed foods you can purchase and are usually loaded with sugars. It is supplemented with vitamins and minerals to make it seem like it's healthy. Because it is sold as a breakfast food, the typical marketing claim is that it is 'loaded with energy'. That's codeword for extra calories that you don't need.

Bread

American bread typically contains refined flour, added sugars, preservatives (like calcium propionate), and dough conditioners (azodicarbonamide). In America, it is closer to a cake than actual bread. Instead opt for sour dough bread from a local bakery. In Australia and New Zealand, breads typically don't have or need preservatives, sugars and the caveat of that is a shorter shelf life.

Cheap yoghurt

Yoghurt is seen as healthy but just like juices, there are many different types of yoghurt. Some yoghurts will want to showcase that they have reduced fat but will compensate with more sugar. Or highlight that they have probiotic cultures but to make them more palatable, will have sugar. Look out for yoghurt that has no sugar added.

Hummus & pre-made dips

Store-bought versions often contain preservatives, stabilisers, and excess salt and oils. Because hummus is a product that doesn't last long without some treatment, preservatives are added to extend its shelf life.

How to read a nutritional label correctly

Nutritional labels are either called the Nutritional Information Panel (NIP) or Nutritional Facts in America and can seem very daunting and cryptic to understand. They have an unfriendly way of showcasing the macronutrients for food and for many people. They are confusing. While they're designed to inform, their perceived complexity often deters the average shopper from giving them more than a passing glance. But understanding these labels is crucial for making informed dietary choices.

No one can be blamed for not wanting to read the label. Even food technologists in the industry have complained that the nutritional information panel is not very intuitive and confuses people. It was almost made to confuse people and steer them away from looking at it. It also doesn't help that each country has their own way of declaring nutrients and ingredients on the pack. However, it is supposed to help people with understanding what they put into their mouths. Here are some tips to look out for on nutritional labels, from a food technologists' perspective.

Let's look at two theoretical products, both packaged as bars for grabbing on the go. Here are the packaging and the nutritional panels. Use this to compare with products you would see on a supermarket shelf.

Goody Oaty Bars

Nutritional Information

Servings per package: 6

Serving size: 40g ——————→ Take note of the serving size

Average quantity per	40g serving	% Daily Intake per serving	100g	
Energy (kJ)	823	9%	2060	Check the amount of energy/calories (divide by 4.2)
Protein (g)	2.7	5%	6.8	
Fat, Total (g)	9.5	14%	23.8	Less than 17.5g per 100g is ideal
-Saturated Fat (g)	5.9	25%	14.8	Less than 5g per 100g is ideal
Carbohydrate (g)	24.9	8%	62.3	
-Sugars (g)	13.9	15%	34.7	Less than 22.5g per 100g is ideal
Sodium (mg)	70	3%	176	Less than 600mg per 100g is ideal

Paul's Protein Bars

Nutritional Information

Servings per package: 5
Serving size: 40g ————————→ Take note of the serving size

Average quantity per	40g serving	% Daily Intake per serving	100g	
Energy (kJ)	828	10%	2070	
Protein (g)	10.1	20%	25.3	This product has high protein quantities
Fat, Total (g)	11.7	17%	29.2	
-Saturated Fat (g)	2.6	11%	6.5	
Carbohydrate (g)	11.3	4%	28.2	
-Sugars (g)	5.6	6%	14.1	
Dietary Fibre (g)	3.9	13%	9.8	Consuming more fibre is generally good for you and has health benefits
Sodium (mg)	146	6%	364	

Goody Oaty Bars and Paul's Protein bars might seem similar at first glance, but they are quite different in terms of the fat, sugar and salt (FSS) content. Goody Oaty bars have more saturated fat and sugar compared to Paul's protein bars. However, the protein bars would be more expensive due to the ingredients contributing to protein and there are less servings in the package.

It's always best to check how many true servings you're really getting on the pack.

Serving size and per 100g

As a food technologist, for my own consumption I typically ignore the daily intake and the serving size column. The serving size was described in the Marketing Tri Factor, from a food technologists and legal perspective, it is a mandatory declaration of a serving size for a food or beverage. However, serving sizes are dictated by the food manufacturer and not always a realistic measure of what a consumer may eat in one sitting. There are some food products where it makes sense that a serving size is the entire product such as single service pouch or punnet yoghurt where you typically consume that in one go. However, something like a chocolate bar or a packet of crisps has a serving size that is not a reflection of how consumers eat them. Some chocolate bars may illustrate what a serving size may look like on a 200g block, which would make it easy to understand what a serving consists of. However, with something like a packet of crisps, most consumers are not going to weigh them out. There are some consumers who could eat an entire 200g of crisps in one sitting.

Instead, opt to focus on the per 100g or 100ml column as this will be more representative of what the food product is composed of. Food technologists typically use this even just for their own calculations and consumption. It's best to think of this as the actual percentage of the food. The per 100g column is a mandatory quantity that all food manufacturers must state on pack.

The Daily Intake (DI)

The daily intake column is an optional line and shown on the nutritional panel when there has been a claim specific to the daily intake. The daily intakes are based on an average adult diet of approximately 8700 kJ or 2080 calories. It serves as a general guide as to how much a nutrient contributes to an 'average' person's total daily diet.

DI's are simplified and rounded reference values and do not serve as individual nutrition advice. The DI's should only be used as a quick comparison and rough guide and not actual advice, because the values are generalised and your energy and nutrient needs are going to be different from these averages. Also, those who have certain health conditions will need to adjust their macro/micronutrients to suit their needs. For example, an office worker may only need 6300 kJ per day while an athlete may need twice as many calories and nutrients than that.

Below are the daily intake values from FSANZ:

Nutrient	Daily intake reference (adult, 8,700 kJ diet)
Energy (kJ)	8700
Protein (g)	50
Fat, Total (g)	70
Saturated Fat (g)	24
Carbohydrate (g)	310
Sugars (g)	90
Dietary Fibre (g)	9.8
Sodium (mg)	2300

Here is a general guide on the high levels to look out for when you're buying food from the supermarket (For specific individual needs, it is recommended to get guidance from a registered dietician):

The recommended daily intake (RDI)

The recommended daily intake (RDI) is the daily intake needed for an adult that is considered to be healthy enough to meet the health requirements of >95% of the population in a particular life stage and gender group. Looking at it objectively, it does have its merits where such a system was supposed to help people understand their nutritional needs and requirements however times have drastically changed. RDIs are more precise and individualised. They are scientific targets and are often used by nutritionists and dieticians as a reference for diet plans and individual nutrition counselling. Not only that, but different countries also have their own equivalent of the RDI system as no one can agree what is needed for the general population. RDI's are not typically placed on the nutritional label as they are for a specific demographic unless the product itself is targeted for a specific type of consumer. Hence why typically only the DI's are used on the labels.

Food Energy – Calories and Kilojoules

Calories and kilojoules are interchangeable as they're measuring the same thing, they just have a different value and name. Like feet and metres, they're both measuring distance but just in different values. However, calories are more commonly used while kilojoules don't roll off the tongue as easily. In America, energy is declared as calories (kcal) and in Australia and New Zealand it is declared in kilojoules(kJ).

Here is how to convert them:

1 kilocalorie (kcal) is equal to 4.2 kilojoules (kJ).

They are units of energy that make our bodies do everything from walking, thinking, running and everything else that you can and can't see. Everything that you do in life requires energy. Just like a car, your body needs fuel. Unlike a car which has just one source of fuel, humans need to get our energy from different sources.

The main different sources of energy are also called MACRONUTRIENTS: There are three types of macronutrients, Protein, Fat and Carbohydrates, aka Carbs.

How does this work in the grand scheme of things?

Your body will start using up fuel that is contained in your body.

Let's say you go for an 8-hour long hike, and you want to pack some goodies in the backpack for fuel. What do you bring?

A carrot

Scroggin or Trail Mix

Chocolate peanut bar

In this case, you want both the scroggin mix and chocolate peanut bar as they will provide you the energy to walk that long trek.

A carrot is great; however, you will use up that energy quickly in the walk. Also, it will weigh quite a bit in the backpack and would be inefficient to bring along as a source of fuel.

Regardless of whether you are going on a hike or having a gym session, you need food as fuel so you can keep going.

The energy density of foods varies for the different types of macronutrients.

For Protein it is 17kJ/g or 4kcal/g

Carbohydrates it is 17kJ/g or 4kcal/g

Fat it is 37kJ/g or 9kcal/g

When it comes to the energy units, make sure not to get confused with calories and kJs. For example, an energy bar from the US may have 250 calories or in Australia energy would have 1045 kJ, which is the same amount of energy.

Protein

Protein is a word associated with bodybuilders and fitness, but it's something that everyone needs. Alongside carbohydrates and fats, protein is one of the three macronutrients that supply energy, support growth, and keep our bodies functioning. Without it, our muscles would weaken, our immune systems would falter, and our bodies would struggle to repair themselves (National Health and Medical Research Council [NHMRC], 2013).

Protein is more than just a buzzword, it is responsible for building and repairing tissues, producing enzymes and hormones, and even supporting immune function (Whitney et al., 2017). But not all proteins are created equal, they are made up of smaller units called **amino acids**, which act like the building blocks of life.

Protein is now the new sweetheart in the food marketing realm and is frequently highlighted on packaging. This is to make it more appealing especially for those who want to get 'gains' or max out their macros, as it is colloquially termed. It is important to know that adequate protein intake is important. However, do take note of the source of protein. Does the protein come from plant or animal sources? Is the protein accompanied with sugar and other flavours to make it more appealing? Unless you're an athlete or highly active individual that requires higher than normal protein amounts, excess protein consumption can lead to kidney strain and stomach pain.

Amino acids aren't all the same, there are **20 different amino acids,** each with unique roles in the body. They are categorised into three groups:

1. **Essential amino acids (EAA)** – Our bodies cannot produce these, so we must get them from food. Without them, vital functions like muscle repair, immune defence, and hormone production would suffer (Wu, 2013).

2. **Conditionally essential amino acids (CEAA)** – Normally, our bodies can make these, but during times of stress, illness, or intense exercise, we may need more from our diet (Hou et al., 2015).
3. **Non-essential amino acids (NEAA)** – These are produced internally, so we don't need to prioritise them in our meals, though they still play important roles in metabolism and overall health.

Here's a quick look at some of the key players:

- **Leucine, Isoleucine & Valine (The Branched Chain AAs also Essential)** – These three essential amino acids are vital for muscle recovery, endurance, and energy during exercise (Shimomura et al., 2006).
- **Lysine (EAA)** – Supports collagen formation, helping maintain strong bones, joints, and skin (Li & Wu, 2018).
- **Tryptophan (EAA)** – Helps with sleep and it also helps regulate mood and growth hormones (Richard et al., 2009).
- **Glutamine (NEAA)** – Fuels gut health and immune function, especially important after intense workouts (Cruzat et al., 2018).
- **Tyrosine (CEAA)** – A precursor to adrenaline and dopamine, helping you stay sharp under stress (Jongkees et al., 2015).

Our bodies can't store amino acids like they do fats or carbs, we need a steady supply from our diet. Animal sources (meat, eggs, dairy) provide all essential amino acids, while plant-based proteins (beans, lentils, quinoa) can also meet needs when combined wisely (NHMRC, 2013). Without enough protein, our bodies would break down muscle for fuel, weaken our immune defences, and slow recovery from injuries. So, whether you're lifting weights or lifting laptops, protein isn't optional, it's essential and more important when you grow older.

Research shows that after age 30, adults lose 3–8% of muscle mass per decade, a process accelerating after 60 (Volpi et al., 2013). This age-related muscle loss, called sarcopenia, increases the risk of frailty, falls, and metabolic slowdown but adequate protein intake can help counteract it (Bauer et al., 2013).

How much protein do you need?

A common guideline is to consume **at least 1 gram of protein per kilogram of body weight daily** (e.g., a 60 kg person would aim for 60g). However, needs vary:

Active individuals may benefit from **1.2–2.2g/kg** to support muscle repair (Jäger et al., 2017).

Older adults (65+) should aim for **1.2–1.5g/kg** to preserve muscle (Deer & Volpi, 2015).

Injury recovery or illness may further increase requirements (Phillips, 2017).

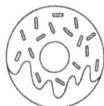

Fat

Fat, also called oil, triglycerides or lipids have been villainised as the culprit causing human diseases in the past. In the 1990s, fat was public enemy number one. Government guidelines, media headlines, and even school cafeterias declared war on dietary fat, blaming it for obesity, heart disease, and soaring cholesterol levels. This fear wasn't baseless, but it was oversimplified, leading to decades of misguided nutrition policies and unintended health consequences.

Food companies capitalised on fat phobia, flooding shelves with "low-fat" products packed with sugar and refined carbs to compensate for lost flavour (Ludwig et al., 2018). We still see products that have the legacy of these claims such as marshmallows, skim milk and crackers which adds to the confusion of consumers when buying products.

Back in the 1990's, the trend was to showcase fat as the big baddie, so the supermarkets were flooded with products that had no fat, low fat, less fat, zero fat. Food marketing was rampantly capitalising on fat phobia in foods. This was shown by products made to have the same taste but with no fat to make them appealing and seem healthy to the consumer. I used to love eating marshmallows when I was a kid because it often had the claim of 99% fat free.

This led to myself and many others eating marshmallows and other products thinking that they were healthy. However, these products were loaded with refined sugar. There were also fat-free ice creams or milk which were essentially tasteless and still taste like milky water (because it kind of is). The fat shaming had taken its toll, and this has led to the confusion that fat was bad. When in high school, I would avoid fatty foods including avocados and peanut butter because they were too fatty. This made my family buy fat free things for a long period of time and probably did some damage to our health, thinking we were doing the best. Now we are more aware about the different types of fats and that they are not all equal, this made me realise that trends and hype need to be diligently checked and scrutinized. Now there are all kinds of 'free' products, and it doesn't always mean it's going to be better or healthier for you.

There was a turning point at around the 2000-2010s where studies showed that populations eating high fat diets rich in nuts, oily fish and olive oil had lower heart disease rates than populations with low-fat diets (Estruch et al., 2013). This coincided with the research and information revealing that refined carbohydrates and sugar were the major drivers of insulin resistance and other metabolic diseases (Lustig, 2013). Pointing the finger at fat has backfired, resulting in products made with excessive sugar causing populations to eat more sugar than they need.

If there is one thing to be clear about, don't villainise ANY macronutrients. Especially fats as they are one of the macronutrients that your body needs. Just like proteins and carbohydrates, not all fats are equal and it's the type of fat that you're consuming that makes a difference.

First let's do some defining of what exactly is fat and its different classes.

Saturated Fats

Sources of saturated fat include coconut oil, butter, lard, cream, cheese and palm oil. Why are saturated fats called saturated? It is because of the molecular structure, it contains single bonds between molecules, which means they can pack more in the small structure as opposed to unsaturated fats which have at least one double bond.

Saturated fats caused a stir in the scientific community on whether they are actually good or bad for you. However, it seems clear that limiting saturated fats in one's diet is best. Excess consumption of saturated fats increases the LDL 'bad' cholesterol which is a major factor in causing cardiovascular disease.

The issue? Saturated fats taste amazing. Foods such as full cream yoghurt, cheese, and ice cream all contain saturated fat and it's easy to overconsume during dinner or dessert time. Saturated fats are usually solid at room temperature due to higher melting points.

Unsaturated fats

Unsaturated fat sources include avocado, nuts, vegetable oil, salmon etc. Unsaturated fats are seen as the great health beacon for those who want an active lifestyle and all the benefits for your head, heart and metabolism. Often referred to as the "good healthy fats," these are found in foods like olive oil, nuts, seeds, and oily fish. Unlike saturated fats, these fats can help lower LDL cholesterol and may reduce blood pressure and inflammation. They're also a key component of heart-healthy diets such as the Mediterranean diet (Mozaffarian et al., 2011).

Yes, if you got this far, this is a subgroup of a subgroup of macronutrients, it's easy to see how consumers can get confused.

Monosaturated fatty acids aka MUFAS

MUFAS have one double bond in their molecular structure. Examples of MUFAS are nuts, olive oil, tallow and sunflower oil.

The benefits of MUFAs are that they may be able to increase HDL 'good' cholesterol and decrease the 'bad' cholesterol. Also replacing MUFA with saturated fats can help with improved insulin sensitivity.

6. The Consumption Tri Factor

Polyunsaturated fatty acids aka PUFAS

You may have heard of Omega 3s and 6s, they are found in fatty fish like salmon, mackerel, flaxseeds, sesame seeds etc. Omega-3s are *anti-inflammatory*, supporting brain function and reducing heart disease risk by lowering triglycerides (Swanson et al., 2012). Omega-6s are *pro-inflammatory* in excess. Modern diets skew heavily toward omega-6s (think processed snacks), disrupting the ideal 1:1 to 1:4 ratio with omega-3s (Simopoulos, 2016).

Trans fat

While saturated fats were wrongly demonised in the 1990s, **trans fats** quietly earned their reputation as the *true* dietary villain and for good reason. Unlike natural fats, artificial trans fats are an industrial byproduct with devastating health effects, leading to global bans and public health warnings. Trans fats are the worst and have consistently shown to be drivers of heart disease and cancer. Stay away from these as much as possible. These are not needed in your body at all. They've been consistently linked to an increased risk of heart disease, stroke, and even certain cancers (Mozaffarian, et al., 2006). While small amounts occur naturally in some animal products, most trans fats are artificially created through a process called hydrogenation. This involves adding hydrogen to vegetable oils to make them more solid and shelf-stable which is ideal for processed foods like margarine, microwave popcorn, and baked goods.

Trans fats (or *trans fatty acids*) are a type of unsaturated fat with an altered chemical structure, making them unnaturally stable and solid at room temperature. They come in two forms:

1. **Natural trans fats** – Found in small amounts in meat and dairy (from ruminant animals like cows). These are *not* strongly linked to harm.
2. **Artificial trans fats** – Created through *hydrogenation*, a process that turns liquid vegetable oils into solid fats (e.g., margarine, shortening). These are the dangerous kind.

Trans fats were everywhere because they are cheap & long-lasting: Ideal for fried foods, baked goods, and processed snacks (think doughnuts, crackers, and fast food). In the 1980s–90s, companies marketed margarine as a "heart-healthy" alternative to butter, despite it being packed with trans fats (Mozaffarian et al., 2006). By the 1990s–2000s, research revealed trans fats to have **raised LDL ("bad") cholesterol and lowered HDL ("good") cholesterol,** a double whammy for heart disease (Willett et al., 1993) and increased inflammation, insulin resistance, and stroke risk (Dhaka et al., 2011).

No safe level exists. Just 2% of daily calories from trans fats (about 4g) raises heart disease risk by 23% (WHO, 2023). Denmark is the first country to ban artificial trans fats in 2003 and it plummeted heart disease deaths (Restrepo & Rieger, 2016). Meanwhile, in Australia and New Zealand, there are voluntary industry reductions, but no full ban yet (FSANZ, 2023).

How to avoid trans fats

Check labels: Look for "partially hydrogenated oils" (now rare in Australia but still in some imported products).

Ditch processed snacks when possible: Opt for whole foods (nuts, seeds, avocado) over packaged biscuits/pastries.

Cook smart: Using olive oil instead of margarine.

Trans fats show that *not all fats are equal*, while the 90s scapegoated natural fats, the real danger lurked in processed foods. Their near eradication is a public health victory, but vigilance remains key.

What is cholesterol?

Everyone has heard of cholesterol, whether it be from your parents, grandparents or just an annoying food advert somewhere. We've all seen the word cholesterol, but most people don't even know what it is. Unfortunately, it's commonly linked with something bad like heart disease. There's a common theme here that too much of a 'good' thing can become detrimental, and this is definitely the case with cholesterol.

Cholesterol is essentially a type of fat that plays an important role in our body, responsible for building, maintaining and regulating cell membranes and hormones to keep you functioning day to day.

As stated before, too much of it is not good. Why?

High levels of cholesterol can cause the narrowing of arteries, which leads to restricting blood flow due to a build-up of fat and/or cholesterol through a process called atherosclerosis. This is where the plaque of fat, white blood cells, cholesterol and other lipids build up on the walls of arteries and hardens. Over time and combined with poor life choices such as not being careful with your diet and neglecting exercise this can lead to a blocked or clotted artery which can lead to a heart attack and ultimately death.

But just like fat, carbohydrates and everything else, not all cholesterol is the same.

There are the different types:

HDL – High density lipoprotein aka the 'Good' cholesterol

HDL cholesterol are like the good cleanup trucks that remove the excess cholesterol from the blood stream and arteries and transport it back to the liver. The liver is like the processing plants for cholesterol, it breaks it down to small parts and gets it out of your body.

LDL – Low density lipoprotein aka the 'Bad' cholesterol

LDL cholesterol is like a delivery truck that takes cholesterol around the body so that they can build cells/membranes etc. Too many delivery trucks on the road or in your blood stream and arteries can cause a traffic artery jam.

6. The Consumption Tri Factor

So, what's the correlation here?

The scientific and medical community find that if you have a higher ratio of Good HDL to Bad LDL cholesterol then your risk of heart disease, stroke etc is reduced.

But here's another factor that comes into play that no one can change.

Your genetics.

Your genetics will determine how your body processes cholesterol. Some simply have high cholesterol genes that run in the family. This is a condition called familial hypercholesterolemia or FH for short. How do you know if you have FH? Get yourself tested. Or if you know that one side of the family has a history of cholesterol related problems such as heart disease, diabetes, stroke etc then you should look out because the percentage of inheriting them from one of your parents is 50%.

It is always best to get yourself tested early for the sake of awareness so you can start making the appropriate lifestyle changes if necessary. A blood test is a good first step of determining what your cholesterol levels are.

So how does cholesterol tie in with the food industry?

Can you imagine the food marketing claims that can run WILD and crazy when consumers don't even know what cholesterol is and all they know or THINK they know is that it has something to do with heart disease?

There was a phase when food companies would make products that sell the idea of lowering cholesterol. That's why you see margarines or certain spreads and oil that state something along the lines of "helps lower cholesterol".

People might jump and immediately assume that this particular brand of oats is all they need to help get rid of their health issues and a future heart attack. While oats *do* contain soluble fibre (which can modestly reduce LDL) (Harvard Health, 2020), many claims exploit consumer confusion.

For countries that do not have strict regulatory bodies, they might get away with it for a period without having to substantiate these claims. Thankfully, in developed countries the laws are a lot stricter, and you see less of this kind of misleading marketing.

Carbohydrates

Carbohydrates or 'Carbs' have been labelled the enemy on numerous fronts for making people fat but if you actually look into it, carbs are not the enemy that the media makes them out to be. Research shows that weight gain occurs primarily due to excessive calorie intake, not carbohydrate intake (Ludwig et al., 2018).

Carbohydrates, just like proteins, also have building blocks. Their building blocks are called saccharides or 'sugars'. Yes, carbohydrates are basically just dense sugars. However, they are an important part of any diet as it's one of the macronutrients that your body needs. They fuel muscles, the central nervous system, and brain function. Critically, they also spare protein from being catabolised for energy, preserving it for muscle repair and growth (Jeukendrup, 2017).

Carbohydrates are predominantly found in whole plant foods: fruits, vegetables, legumes, and grains. These provide not just energy but also fibre, phytonutrients, and essential micronutrients (Slavin, 2013).

Carbohydrates are classified into **simple** (rapidly absorbed) and **complex** (slow digesting) based on their chemical structure:

The key difference between a simple and complex carbohydrate is down to the chemical structure at a molecular level, and also how quickly the sugars the carbohydrates contain are broken down and absorbed by the body.

Simple carbohydrates contain one or two sugar molecules such as fructose which are found in fruit. Fruit by itself does contain simple sugars, however it is accompanied with vitamins and minerals that your body needs. Refined sugars in coke and sweets are processed to the point where they are easily absorbed by the body leading to weight gain and contain little to no vitamins or minerals (Malik & Hu, 2022).

Complex carbohydrates also known as polysaccharides would have three or more sugar molecules and these are found in the more 'starchy' carb foods that we love to hate or eat such as bread, pasta, noodles, potatoes etc. Complex carbs will break down into sugars regardless; however, they provide sustained energy in the long run and reduce hunger fluctuations (Augustin et al., 2015).

So why did carbs get the bad rep? Let's take a look at what they do in your body.

Once the carbohydrates have been broken up into sugar molecules, they are absorbed by the small intestine and go into your bloodstream and into the liver. The liver converts these sugars into glucose with a tag partner called insulin that transports them to other parts of the body that require energy for physical activity and bodily functions.

Sometimes your body doesn't need the glucose so it will tuck it away in the skeletal muscles in a form called glycogen or in the liver. However, once these slots are full, the excess carbs are then stored as fat (Frayn, 2010).

Just like fat, there are 'Good' and 'Bad' carbs. And there are several ways of looking into it, one of them is the GI or the Glycaemic Index. Many people find this hard to grasp however it's easy once you understand it. The glycaemic index is an indication of how quickly the carbohydrate is absorbed in your body. Foods that have carbs are often categorised as either 'Low' GI and never 'High' Gi. Why?

6. The Consumption Tri Factor

High GI foods are ones that are absorbed quickly causing blood glucose levels to rise faster. This is usually simple carbohydrates and many UPF are typically high GI.

Examples of high GI foods include honey, refined sugar such as white sugar, fruit juices, white bread.

Low GI foods take more time to be digested and have slower absorption compared to their high GI counterparts and consist of complex carbohydrates.

Examples of low GI foods include whole grain bread, beans, legumes, and brown rice.

The difference between High and Low GI foods are as below:

High GI Simple Carbs

- Lots of energy/High in calories

- Little to no nutrients

- Little to no fibre

- Is often accompanied with saturated fats

Low GI Complex Carbs

- High in fibre

- Usually has vitamins and minerals

- Has a moderate amount of calories

- Give sustained energy

- Usually accompanied with low fat content

Carbs are the primary source of energy that your body uses and if you lead an active lifestyle, this needs to be replenished on a frequent basis. However, if you live a sedentary lifestyle, you don't need so many carbohydrates as they contain energy that will be stored as fat. Carbs and sugars are not the same thing, but carbs are just big blocks of sugar lumped together to help you get through the day!

Fibre

What exactly is fibre? It helps when you go 'poo' and keeps you regular. Is it the same as carbohydrates? Almost but not quite, the biggest difference is that it cannot be digested by the small intestine of our bodies.

Fibre or dietary fibre as it's also called is commonly found in plants such as fruits, vegetables, whole grains and legumes. Dietary fibre consists of non-digestible carbohydrates that are resistant to absorption and digestion.

You would have heard numerous health outlets about eating more fibre and it certainly has its benefits. From a food technologist's point of view, fibre is truly beneficial because it reduces your risk of heart disease, diabetes and helps with relieving constipation. It isn't a made-up gimmick to simply try and sell more things to the consumer. Certain products such as dried fruit, cereal and bread products love claiming that they are a source of fibre because fibre has a positive health association with it even if the consumer doesn't exactly know what it is.

A great example of a fibre boosting food is prunes. The shrivelled dried plum is a great snack that can be taken everywhere and is known for 'keeping you regular'.

Prunes do have a good amount of fibre in them and if you are constipated, prune juice is a great natural way to let loose.

Looking at dietary fibre, again there are different types.

Fibre can be classified as soluble which means it dissolves in water or insoluble fibre which means it does not dissolve in water.

Soluble fibre

This type of fibre dissolves in water and can be prebiotic. It helps you feel full for longer from delaying how long food stays in the stomach and improving glycaemic control (Brown et al., 2019). It can help lower blood cholesterol and glucose levels. Soluble fibre is found in legumes, oats, peas, nuts, artichokes, quinoa, prunes, avocados, carrots, barley and psyllium.

Insoluble fibre

Insoluble fibre does not dissolve in water.

This type of fibre helps ease the movement of material through your digestive system and increases stool bulk by absorbing water as it passes through the digestive system (Dahl & Stewart, 2015). Insoluble fibre can also be a prebiotic.

Sources of insoluble dietary fibre include seeds, nuts, beans, potato skin, zucchini/courgette, celery, green beans and peas.

The best way to get the most types of fibre is to eat a variety of high fibre plant-based foods as the amount of soluble and insoluble fibre will vary in different plant foods.

The benefits of a high-fibre diet:

They are numerous but let's start with the benefit of keeping you regular.

How does it do this?

Dietary fibre helps soften and increase the weight of your stool. If you have watery stool, then fibre helps by bulking it up through absorbing water so that it is easier to pass through your system. Likewise, if you have small stools, fibre will bulk it up making it easier to pass. Insoluble fibre is responsible for doing this as it hastens the road for food to go through your digestive system.

6. The Consumption Tri Factor

A high-fibre diet has many benefits, which include:

- Helps maintain bowel health. A high-fibre diet may lower your risk of developing haemorrhoids and small pouches in your colon (diverticular disease). Some fibre is fermented in the colon. Researchers are looking at how this may play a role in preventing diseases of the colon (Crowe et al., 2011).

- Lowers cholesterol levels. Soluble fibre found in beans, oats, flaxseed and oat bran may help lower total blood cholesterol levels by lowering low-density lipoprotein, or "bad," cholesterol levels. Studies also have shown that high-fibre foods may have other heart-health benefits, such as reducing blood pressure and inflammation (Wanders et al., 2011).

- Helps control blood sugar levels. In people with diabetes, soluble fibre can slow the absorption of sugar and help improve blood sugar levels. A healthy diet that includes insoluble fibre may also reduce the risk of developing type 2 diabetes (Weickert & Pfeiffer, 2018).

- Aids in achieving healthy weight. High-fibre foods tend to be more filling than low-fibre foods, so you're likely to eat less and stay satisfied longer. And high-fibre foods tend to take longer to eat and to be less "energy dense," which means they have fewer calories for the same volume of food.

Carbohydrates are essential and the problem lies in overconsumption of processed carbs, not whole-food sources. By choosing low-GI, fibre-rich options, you can fuel your body effectively without guilt.

Conclusion: The Consumption Tri Factor

When I was a 10-year-old kid, McDonalds used to have Big Mac specials where you could get 4 Big Macs for $10. This is a great deal especially if you love Big Macs. Also don't forget, Big Macs were actually big in the 90s and for a 10-year-old, one burger is more than a half a day's calories in one serving.

As a treat, my parents would buy four Big Macs for me every weekend. Probably to shut me up and because I kept asking for it (this was the irresistible tri factor kicking in). My parents were also convinced by the convenience, price and taste of the Big Mac deal. It got to a point where I got sick of eating so many Big Macs and it was a turning point in my life even at a young age. When my parents offered it almost every weekend, it felt like a cop out from their end. I could feel that it was affecting my health, and I was becoming overweight as a child. I started to become the fat kid in school, and I knew deep down that this wasn't sustainable.

I started to crave more home cooked meals that my mother made instead. The excess consumption of the Irresistible Tri Factor made me revolt against fast food for a long time, as if I had done my own 'Supersize me' experiment before it became a thing. This is the perfect example of the consumption tri factor working in the context of a family looking to feed hungry children. This is a situation that many families face daily.

Fast food and certain ultra processed foods are seen as the solution because it is super convenient, tasty enough to satisfy the family taste buds and reasonably affordable. Combine that with the irresistible tri factor and from a food industry perspective, you have the perfect customer that will keep coming back.

Becoming a Food Detective: Your Practical Toolkit – For Foods Sake!

Understanding macronutrients is crucial, but knowledge alone isn't power without action.

This is where you step into the role of a true Food Detective. Forget passive shopping; it's time to actively investigate using the three key investigative lenses: **Irresistible (Fat, Sugar, Salt), Marketing** and **Consumption.** Arm yourself with scepticism and curiosity by doing the following:

1. Crack the Irresistible Tri Factor: Fat, Sugar, Salt (FSS) Processed foods often hijack our taste buds with potent combinations of fat, sugar, and salt (Moss, 2013) as stated in the previous chapters. Your nutritional panel is your best guide and focus on the **per 100g column** for the most informative comparisons:

- **The FSS Factor:** How much total fat, sugar, and salt (sodium) does it contain?
- Be particularly alert for products high in *all three*, this is the classic "irresistible" formula designed for overconsumption (Monteiro, Cannon, Levy, et al., 2019).
- **Drill down on the irresistible tri factor:** Specifically, how much is saturated fat? How much is sugar? How much is salt? These details matter for health.
- **Serving size sleuthing:** While the 100g column is your baseline, do glance at the serving size. If one tiny serving delivers a massive hit of FSS (say, over half your daily limit for one element), question why it needs to be so potent. Is it masking low-quality ingredients? Is it there for taste, mouthfeel?
- **Ingredient Intel:** The ingredients list tells the *real* story, in descending order by weight.

First ingredient clue: If sugar (or a synonym like sucrose, fructose, syrup) is the *first* ingredient in something not explicitly a sweet treat (like a pasta sauce or "healthy" snack bar), be very wary.

Don't be scared of the unfamiliar (But question it): While not all E-numbers or chemical names are harmful, their presence indicates processing. Ask: Why is this additive here? Is it for preservation, artificial colour, flavour enhancement, or texture? Could this food exist in a recognisable form without them?

Consider the degree of processing, is the original food matrix still intact or completely destroyed?

2. Decipher the Marketing Maze: See Beyond the Glitter

Food packaging is a carefully crafted sales pitch. Your first detective skill is seeing through it. Ask yourself:

- **Strip back the shine:** Mentally remove the logos, vibrant colours, and alluring graphics. What remains? View it objectively as a packaged *product*, not a promise of health or happiness. Recognise that branding often prioritises recognition over nutritional quality (Harris, Pomeranz, Lobstein, & Brownell, 2009).

- **Function over fluff:** Is the packaging genuinely necessary to protect the food, or is it excessive, designed purely to catch your eye and justify a higher price? Call out unnecessary layers and wasteful design.

- **Typography tells a tale:** What feeling does the font style evoke (rustic, futuristic, "healthy")? Is this emotional cue distracting you from scrutinising what's actually *inside*? If you're tempted *just* because it looks appealing, put it down.

- **Shop smart, not fast:** Go armed with a list. Pause. Ask: "Do I genuinely *need* this product, or just *this brand's version* of it?" Compare alternatives calmly and not in a state of hunger.

- **Value vs. Vanity:** Check the price per 100g or per kilogram. Be astounded by the range! A basic muesli might be $5 per 400g pack, while a heavily marketed one hits $20 for the same weight. Do the taste, ingredients, or *actual* quality justify that difference, or are you paying for the marketing story and fancy box? What is the realistic serving size, and is it easy to measure out?

3. Assess the Consumption Realities: Packaging, Price, Flavours & NIP

Evaluate the practicalities and true value proposition:

- **Flavour Fakery or the Real Deal?** Does the flavour (e.g., "luscious strawberry") come from actual strawberries high on the ingredients list, or is it conjured up with "natural flavours" and a dash of colour (124)? Be sceptical of vibrant pictures not backed by real ingredients.

- **Additive accountability:** Refer to the ingredients list. What additives are present? Look up their function (preservative, colour, emulsifier, flavour enhancer). Ask yourself if their presence is justified for safety or function, or merely for cosmetic appeal or shelf-life extension at the cost of whole ingredients.

- **The "Could I Make This?" test:** Is this a simple combination of ingredients you could realistically prepare in your kitchen (like a basic soup or hummus)? Or is it a highly engineered product requiring industrial processes you couldn't replicate? If it's the latter, does that processing offer a *genuine* benefit (like a safe, convenient, nutritious option), or just an artificial texture or extreme shelf-life?

- **Who's behind the brand?** Is it a multinational giant, a small local producer, or a supermarket's own label? This can sometimes influence priorities (profit margins vs. niche quality), though it's not a guaranteed indicator – investigate the actual product.

- **Price point justification:** Does the price truly reflect the quality and quantity of the ingredients inside? Are you paying for premium components (like extra virgin olive oil, organic nuts, free-range meat), the convenient packaging and ethical sourcing, or mostly for marketing, excessive packaging, and brand hype? Let the ingredients and nutritional value be your guide, not the price tag alone.

- **Food or product?** Ask yourself, when you're purchasing any food, are you purchasing a food for nutrients or a product designed to give you the Irresistible Tri Factor?

By consciously applying these three investigative lenses – **Marketing, Irresistible (FSS),** and **Consumption,** you move from being a passive consumer to an empowered Food Detective. You'll make choices based on evidence, not illusion, taking control of what fuels your body.

Moderation and Balance

What is moderation?

You've likely heard the phrase "everything in moderation." But what does that truly mean for *your* plate, your body, and your life? It's often tossed around casually, perhaps after indulging in one too many doughnuts or chocolates. Then there's the confounding twist: "everything in moderation, *including* moderation." No wonder many feel lost navigating what "moderation" even looks like amidst aisles of processed and ultra-processed foods.

Ask yourself: **What do YOU truly want to achieve?**

Consider your lifestyle goals, dietary needs, and taste preferences. Imagine a spectrum: Impoverished > Malnourished > Imbalance > Moderation > Overspill > Excess > Gluttony

Many find themselves oscillating between **Imbalance** and **Overspill**. Perhaps you're not eating enough fresh produce, a widespread issue linked to insufficient dietary fibre (Australian Bureau of Statistics, 2018). Maybe your culinary world feels limited, confined by cultural exposure. You might feel perpetually sub-optimal, unaware that low-grade inflammation could be the culprit (Furman et al., 2019).

Finding Your moderation: The Mind-Body Connection

The key to unlocking moderation lies in understanding a fundamental truth often overlooked: your mind and body are not separate entities; they are one interconnected system. As neuroscientist Antonio Damasio (1994) elegantly argued, our minds are deeply embodied. This is why the adage "You are what you eat" resonates with profound accuracy. The food you consume directly shapes your physical state *and* your mental landscape.

Modern life often severs this connection. We've become increasingly sedentary, paying for exercise because our daily routines lack movement (World Health Organization, 2020). Crushing workloads, digital immersion, and the lure of instant gratification led us to neglect our physical vessels. We often treat our bodies merely as containers for our thoughts, ignoring their signals until illness strikes. Our ancestors across cultures inherently understood the vital link nurtured by mindful eating and movement.

Please don't wait for disease to appreciate your current wellness.

Listen to your body's intelligence

Take my experience: I'm lactose sensitive. Consuming feta cheese, the one cheese my body vehemently rejects, is a guaranteed recipe for a derailed day. Bloating sets in, my brain fixates on the discomfort, mood plummets, and my focus evaporates. This seemingly small reaction underscores a powerful reality: your gut and brain are in constant, intimate conversation (Carabotti et al., 2015). Unhealthy foods offer fleeting pleasure but extract a hidden tax. Your body strains under the overload of excess calorie and the Irresistible Tri Factor of fat, sugar, and salt. The consequences are inflammation, metabolic dysfunction, mood shifts, and might simmer for years before erupting (Monteiro et al., 2019). Our physiology hasn't evolved to match our modern, processed diets. Here's how to tap into that intelligence with this exercise:

How do you train for that mental discipline? There are several approaches, the best way is to take the time and appreciate the taste, texture, aromas, flavours, and mouthfeel of what you're eating as opposed to just scoffing it down.

🔍 **Food detectives exercise!**

Try this to appreciate foods and mental discipline

Take a grape. One single grape.

Using your fingers just look at the shape, colour and feel the skin around it. Note how it feels on your fingers.

Smell it, ask yourself what does it smell like? Can you smell the individual notes of sweetness or earthiness?

Put it in your mouth and leave it there for 20 seconds. Do not chew. This is going to feel weird and you'd want to spit it out or bite into it straight away.

After 20 seconds, take one slow bite and notice how the juice and flesh spill out onto your tongue.

Then 5 more bites and observe in your mouth how it becomes softer and smaller until it is completely gone.

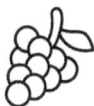

Why do this exercise? It shows just how much we simply just throw something in our mouths, do the mandatory chews so the food goes down our throats without truly appreciating food as it is.

This is a simple yet crucial exercise - food is something that should be celebrated and enjoyed.

6. The Consumption Tri Factor

It can be done for simple foods or your meals at expensive restaurants - it can be done at any time.

Slowing down your eating and slowing down your mind so that it can process and understand what is happening.

Another part of mental discipline is knowing how to evaluate/approximate whether a food will contain more protein, carbohydrates, sugars etc before taking a bite. For a packaged good, just look at the nutritional information.

The System and the Tri Factor Trap

Certain industries capitalise on the widespread misunderstanding of the mind-body-food connection. They target vulnerable groups, glorifying convenient, hyper-palatable foods meticulously engineered to hit the irresistible tri factor" but lacking nutrition (Gearhardt et al., 2011). Clever marketing sells a lifestyle, not sustenance. Nutrient-poor options are often cheaper and more accessible than whole foods, creating a pernicious trap. It fosters the belief that taste is the *only* valid reason to eat, marginalising nourishment.

It's a sticky web of ignorance, difficult to escape. Remember Jamie Oliver's attempt to bring food education to disadvantaged US students? His project faced resistance and was cut short (Oliver, 2010). Those children, with limited access to fresh food or nutritional knowledge, were caught in a cycle: poor diet hindering concentration and learning, limiting future prospects, and perpetuating disadvantage across generations. It's a form of unseen enslavement to a system designed for profit, not health. While not universal, such practices are documented, particularly in systems prioritising cheap calories over nutritional value (Nestle, 2013).

The Non-Negotiable Partner: Exercise

Even with perfect eating, a crucial element completes the pursuit of health: **Exercise.** It's no longer optional for wellbeing, yet many dismiss it as inconvenient, painful, or a waste of time. Without movement, our bodies age faster, metabolism slows, and the mind-body connection weakens. Exercise builds resilience, stronger muscles, a robust immune system, sustained energy, and enhanced mental clarity (Mikkelsen et al., 2017). It directly combats inflammation and improves mood regulation. The rewards aren't instant like a doughnut's sugar rush; they accrue steadily, requiring discipline.

This delayed gratification is often the hurdle.

Common attitudes blocking movement include:

- Prioritising food pleasure over physical effort.
- Viewing exercise as pointless vanity.
- Perceiving a lack of time or energy.
- Finding physical exertion socially "uncool" in some cultures.

This mindset needs shifting. Barring genuine health limitations, incorporating movement is essential.

It doesn't mean you need to be at the gym all the time, instead find *your* joy through movement like dancing, hiking, swimming, team sports, yoga, or whatever you enjoy. Start, observe how you feel *afterwards*, the endorphin lift, the clarity. Initial discomfort means your body is adapting, growing stronger. Discovering an activity you love transforms exercise from chore to cherished ritual. Your future self will thank you for the investment.

Become the detective: Integrating the Tri Factors

Finding true moderation isn't passive. It demands becoming a Food Detective, consciously integrating your shopping lens with the Marketing, Consumption and Irresistible Tri Factors.

By investigating these elements within yourself and your environment, you move beyond simplistic sayings into empowered, personalised balance. It's about reclaiming agency over your wellbeing, one conscious choice at a time.

What is improving in the food industry?

The Australian and New Zealand food industry is making tangible strides toward greater transparency and sustainability. A significant development is the move to make the Health Star Rating (HSR) system compulsory on packaged foods. This initiative empowers consumers to make informed choices by standardising nutritional comparisons at a glance (Food Standards Australia New Zealand [FSANZ],

2023). Concurrently, wholefoods are becoming more accessible, aided by innovations in food processing and distribution that preserve nutritional integrity while extending shelf life.

Sustainability has been a core focus for major manufacturers with recyclable packaging rapidly becoming the norm, driven by both consumer demand and supermarket policies requiring it for shelf placement (Australian Food and Grocery Council [AFGC], 2022). Beyond recycling, companies are investing in breakthrough biodegradable materials, such as plant-based films and edible coatings, to reduce plastic waste.

Transparency is also rising. Plain English Allergen Labelling (PEAL) initiatives encourage clearer ingredient lists, while brands increasingly disclose sourcing and production methods. This shift addresses growing consumer demand for authenticity.

Addressing Misconceptions:
Common misunderstandings about food processing persist. For instance, UHT (shelf-stable) milk remains nutritionally comparable to fresh milk, ultra-high-temperature processing simply extends shelf life without additives. Long life milk requires heat processing to ensure that it is safe in the long run, especially the milk products in the tetrapak. These milk products have the advantage of being shelf stable and don't need any other additives as they have been made commercially sterile and can usually last more than

a year. This is still milk and it's a convenient way of getting milk when you don't have a fresh option and it doesn't have any additives.

Similarly, instant coffee is purely roasted coffee beans subjected to extraction and drying; no "chemical additives" are needed. These processes reflect food science, not artificial manipulation (McClements, 2020).

Areas for Growth: Where the industry must aim higher
Despite progress, critical gaps remain. Marketing transparency needs urgent attention. While packaging claims like "natural" or "no added sugar" abound, they often mislead, such as honey labelled "no added sugar" (honey *is* sugar) or plant-based snacks implying health benefits despite high processing levels. Tighter regulation of on-pack claims and imagery is essential, particularly for smaller producers where oversight is inconsistent (Lawrence et al., 2022).

The industry also falls short in leveraging food waste. Vast quantities of edible by-products (e.g., fruit pulps, spent grains) are discarded rather than upcycled into ingredients or biofuels, a missed economic and environmental opportunity (CSIRO, 2021).

Nutritional information panels (NIPs) remain overwhelming for many shoppers. Simplifying their format and mandating clear explanations of additives (e.g., "citric acid: a preservative derived from citrus fruits") would demystify labels and counter misleading marketing.

Finally, the pursuit of fleeting flavour trends often prioritises novelty over nutrition or genuine culinary value. Redirecting this innovation toward nutrient-dense, minimally processed options would better serve public health. Crucially, the notion that "processed equals non-food" is scientifically inaccurate, techniques like freezing, fermenting, or canning preserve food safety and nutrition. The real issue lies in *ultra-*processing, where certain additives, refining and the transforming of the food matrix diminish health value (Monteiro et al., 2019).

Conclusion

Processed food and ultra processed food have a place in our lives, but they shouldn't dominate. Now that you know about the Irresistible, Marketing and Consumption Tri Factors I hope that you get an objective view on how processed food is made, marketed, packed, distributed and consumed.

If anything, I hope that you realise that you have more control over what you put in your mouth and appreciate that what we take for granted in terms of the food we purchase and consume is and should be more than just a 'product'. Most of these products have been created to ensure that you the consumer has a great experience, can eat it safely and of course, eat it again.

Understanding how processed foods can contribute positively to your lifestyle and diet is a process that takes patience, time, money and open tastebuds. Being wary, objective and aware of how marketing is being used to manipulate consumers to purchase something that is deemed better for you when it's not, is a powerful tool to help you and your family make better choices.

As a former food technologist, I covered as much as I could for this first book. There is more to cover when it comes to food as I could go on forever.

Conclusion

Remember, regardless if it's fresh or processed food, look to being a conscious consumer and a food detective who isn't lured into buying something just because it tastes great or has the Irresistible Tri Factor and you will actually enjoy consuming it because it has a purpose in your life.

For food's sake, consume wisely, with your own balanced moderation that allows you to live your best life.

References

The definition of food, processed food and ultra processed food

Forde, C. G., et al. (2013). Oral processing characteristics of solid savoury meal components. *Food Quality and Preference, 28*(1), 116-126.

Hall, K. D., et al. (2019). Ultra-processed diets cause excess calorie intake and weight gain. *Cell Metabolism, 30*(1), 67-77.

Marco, M. L., Heeney, D., Binda, S., Cifelli, C. J., Cotter, P. D., Foligné, B., Gänzle, M., Kort, R., Pasin, G., Pihlanto, A., Smid, E. J., & Hutkins, R. (2017). Health benefits of fermented foods: Microbiota and beyond. *Current Opinion in Biotechnology, 44*, 94-102. https://doi.org/10.1016/j.copbio.2016.11.010

Monteiro, C. A., et al. (2019). Ultra-processed foods: What they are and how to identify them. *Public Health Nutrition, 22*(5), 936–941.

The entire process of making a food product

Cooper, R. G. (2019). The drivers of success in new-product development. *Industrial Marketing*

References

Management, 76, 36-47. https://doi.org/10.1016/j.indmarman.2018.07.005

Floros, J. D., et al. (2010). Feeding the world today and tomorrow: The importance of food science and technology. *Comprehensive Reviews in Food Science and Food Safety, 9*(1), 572-599. https://doi.org/10.1111/j.1541-4337.2010.00127.x

Hobbs, J. E., & Young, L. M. (2022). *The economics of private label foods and beverages.* Springer.

The Irresistible Tri Factor

Fat

Lichtenstein, A. H., Ausman, L. M., Jalbert, S. M., & Schaefer, E. J. (1999). Effects of different forms of dietary hydrogenated fats on serum lipoprotein cholesterol levels. *New England Journal of Medicine, 340*(25), 1933–1940. https://doi.org/10.1056/NEJM199906243402502

Mozaffarian, D., Katan, M. B., Ascherio, A., Stampfer, M. J., & Willett, W. C. (2006). Trans fatty acids and cardiovascular disease. *New England Journal of Medicine, 354*(15), 1601–1613. https://doi.org/10.1056/NEJMra054035

Mozaffarian, D., Micha, R., & Wallace, S. (2011). Effects on coronary heart disease of increasing polyunsaturated fat in place of saturated fat: A systematic review and meta-analysis of randomized controlled trials. *PLoS Medicine, 7*(3), e1000252. https://doi.org/10.1371/journal.pmed.1000252

St-Onge, M. P., & Jones, P. J. H. (2002). Physiological effects of medium-chain triglycerides: Potential agents in the prevention of obesity. *Journal of Nutrition, 132*(3), 329–332. https://doi.org/10.1093/jn/132.3.329

Sugar

Avena, N. M., Rada, P., & Hoebel, B. G. (2008). *Evidence for sugar addiction: Behavioral and neurochemical effects of intermittent, excessive sugar intake.* Neuroscience & Biobehavioral Reviews, 32(1), 20–39. https://doi.org/10.1016/j.neubiorev.2007.04.019

Bliss, T. (2010). *The End of Overeating: Taking Control of the Insatiable American Appetite.* Rodale Books.

DiFeliceantonio, A. G., et al. (2012). *Nucleus accumbens opioid receptors mediate the formation of Pavlovian associations between fat-predictive cues and fat ingestion.* Journal of Neuroscience, 32(20), 7025–7030. https://doi.org/10.1523/JNEUROSCI.6461-11.2012

Galloway, J. H. (2005). *The Sugar Cane Industry: An Historical Geography from Its Origins to 1914.* Cambridge University Press.

Gearhardt, A. N., et al. (2011). *Can food be addictive? Public health and policy implications.* Addiction, 106(7), 1208–1212. https://doi.org/10.1111/j.1360-0443.2010.03301.x

References

Gropper, S. S., & Smith, J. L. (2021). *Advanced nutrition and human metabolism* (8th ed.). Cengage Learning.

Lenoir, M., Serre, F., Cantin, L., & Ahmed, S. H. (2007). *Intense sweetness surpasses cocaine reward.* PLoS One, 2(8), e698. https://doi.org/10.1371/journal.pone.0000698

Ludwig, D. S., & Ebbeling, C. B. (2018). *The Carbohydrate-Insulin Model of Obesity: Beyond "Calories In, Calories Out".* JAMA Internal Medicine, 178(8), 1098–1103. https://doi.org/10.1001/jamainternmed.2018.2933

World Health Organization. (2015). *Guideline: Sugars intake for adults and children.* https://www.who.int/publications/i/item/9789241549028

Salt

American Heart Association. (2021). *How much sodium should I eat per day?* https://www.heart.org/en/healthy-living/healthy-eating/eat-smart/sodium/how-much-sodium-should-i-eat-per-day

Appel, L. J., Frohlich, E. D., Hall, J. E., Pearson, T. A., Sacco, R. L., Seals, D. R., ... & Van Horn, L. V. (2011). The importance of population-wide sodium reduction as a means to prevent cardiovascular disease and stroke: a call to action from the American Heart Association. *Circulation*, 123(10), 1138–1143. https://doi.org/10.1161/CIR.0b013e31820d0793

He, F. J., Brinsden, H. C., & MacGregor, G. A. (2013). Salt reduction in the United Kingdom: a successful experiment in public health. *Journal of Human Hypertension*, 28(6), 345–352. https://doi.org/10.1038/jhh.2013.105

Kurlansky, M. (2002). *Salt: A world history*. Walker & Company.

Mouthfeel

Spence, C. (2015). *Eating with our ears: assessing the importance of the sounds of consumption on our perception and enjoyment of multisensory flavour experiences*. Flavour, 4(1), 3.

Public Health Collaboration. (2022). *Ultra-Processed Foods: A Definition For Public Health*.

Witherly, S. A. (2007). *Why Humans Like Junk Food*. iUniverse.

How the Irresistible Tri Factor caused so much strife in the world

Kessler, D. A. (2009). *The end of overeating: Taking control of the insatiable American appetite*. Rodale Books.

Moodie, R., Stuckler, D., Monteiro, C., Sheron, N., Neal, B., Thamarangsi, T., Lincoln, P., & Casswell, S. (2013). Profits and pandemics: Prevention of harmful effects of tobacco, alcohol, and ultra-processed food and drink industries. *The Lancet, 381*(9867), 670–679. https://doi.org/10.1016/S0140-6736(12)62089-3

What are additives and are they that scary?

FSANZ (2019). *Food Additives Numerical List.*

EFSA (2021). *Re-evaluation of Food Additives.*

Salt, L.P. (2020). *Flavor Enhancement in Processed Foods. J. Food Sci.*

How food processing works

Floros, J. D., et al. (2010). Feeding the world today and tomorrow: The importance of food science and technology. *Comprehensive Reviews in Food Science and Food Safety, 9*(1), 572–599.

Monteiro, C. A., et al. (2019). Ultra-processed foods: What they are and how to identify them. *Public Health Nutrition, 22*(5), 936–941.

What's the deal with emulsifiers?

EFSA Panel on Food Additives. (2017). *Re-evaluation of lecithins (E 322) as a food additive.* EFSA Journal, 15(4), 4742. https://doi.org/10.2903/j.efsa.2017.4742

Sellem, L., Srour, B., Javaux, G., et al. (2023). *Food additive emulsifiers and risk of cardiovascular disease.*

BMJ, 382, e076058. https://doi.org/10.1136/bmj-2023-076058

Sensory Science

Berridge, K. C., & Kringelbach, M. L. (2015). Pleasure systems in the brain. *Neuron, 86*(3), 646-664. https://doi.org/10.1016/j.neuron.2015.02.018

Kemp, S. E., Hollowood, T., & Hort, J. (2018). *Sensory evaluation: A practical handbook*. Wiley.

Lawless, H. T., & Heymann, H. (2010). *Sensory evaluation of food: Principles and practices* (2nd ed.). Springer.

Supertaster

Duffy, V. B., Davidson, A. C., Kidd, J. R., Kidd, K. K., Speed, W. C., Pakstis, A. J., … & Bartoshuk, L. M. (2004). Bitter receptor gene (TAS2R38), 6-n-propylthiouracil (PROP) bitterness and alcohol intake. *Alcoholism: Clinical and Experimental Research, 28*(11), 1629-1637. https://doi.org/10.1097/01.ALC.0000145789.55183.D4

Hayes, J. E., Wallace, M. R., Knopik, V. S., Herbstman, D. M., Bartoshuk, L. M., & Duffy, V. B. (2011). Allelic variation in TAS2R bitter receptor genes associates with variation in sensations from ingestive behaviors toward common bitter beverages in adults. *Chemical Senses, 36*(3), 311-319. https://doi.org/10.1093/chemse/bjq132

References

How Food Marketers view consumers

Andrews, J. C., Netemeyer, R. G., & Burton, S. (2011). Consumer generalization of nutrient content claims in advertising. Journal of Marketing.

Elliott, C. (2012). Marketing foods to children: Are we "pestering" parents? Public Health Nutrition.

Harris, J. L., et al. (2009). Priming effects of television food advertising on eating behaviour. Health Psychology.

Hieke, S., et al. (2016). Nutritional puffery in food marketing. Appetite.

Moodie, R., et al. (2013). The commercial determinants of health. The Lancet.

Nestle, M. (2018). Unsavory Truth: How Food Companies Skew the Science of What We Eat. Basic Books.

Pollan, M. (2008). In Defense of Food: An Eater's Manifesto. Penguin Press.

Scrinis, G. (2013). Nutritionism: The Science and Politics of Dietary Advice. Columbia University Press

What determines what food product you buy: budget, how you buy a food product (lifestyle, health, stage in life, budget, location, culture, occasion, time, values etc)

Ampuero, O., & Vila, N. (2006). Consumer perceptions of product packaging. Journal of Consumer Marketing, 23(2), 100-112. https://doi.org/10.1108/07363760610655032

Appadurai, A. (1996). *Modernity at large: Cultural dimensions of globalization.* University of Minnesota Press.

Belk, R. W. (1988). "Possessions and the Extended Self."

Chandon, P., Hutchinson, J. W., Bradlow, E. T., & Young, S. H. (2009). Does in-store marketing work? Effects of the number and position of shelf facings on brand attention and evaluation at the point of purchase. Journal of Marketing, 73(6), 1-17. https://doi.org/10.1509/jmkg.73.6.1

Douglas, M., & Isherwood, B. (1979). The world of goods: Towards an anthropology of consumption. Basic Books.

Haws, K. L., & Bearden, W. O. (2006). Dynamic pricing and consumer fairness perceptions. Journal of Consumer Research, 33(2), 304–311. https://doi.org/10.1086/508435

Johnston, J., & Szabo, M. (2011). Reflexivity and the Whole Foods Market consumer: The lived experience of shopping for change. Agriculture and Human Values, 28(3), 303-319. https://doi.org/10.1007/s10460-010-9283-9

References

Walker, R. E., Block, K. M., & Correa, J. (2010). Disparities and access to healthy food in the United States: A review of food deserts literature. *Health & Place,* *16*(5), 876–884. https://doi.org/10.1016/j.healthplace.2010.04.013

The Role of Branding in Food Marketing

Aaker, D. A. (1996). *Building Strong Brands.* Free Press.

Howard, P. H. (2016). *Concentration and Power in the Food System.* Bloomsbury.

Kapferer, J. N. (2012). *The New Strategic Brand Management.* Kogan Page.

Keller, K. L. (2013). *Strategic Brand Management.* Pearson.

Nestle, M. (2018). *Unsavory Truth: How Food Companies Skew the Science of What We Eat.* Basic Books.

Scrinis, G. (2013). *Nutritionism: The Science and Politics of Dietary Advice.* Columbia University Press.

Wansink, B. (2006). *Mindless Eating: Why We Eat More Than We Think.* Bantam.

Knowing what is the marketing that is distracting and what is going to be useful

Aaker, D. A. (1996). Building Strong Brands. Free Press.

Keller, K. L. (2013). Strategic Brand Management. Pearson.

Pollan, M. (2008). In Defense of Food: An Eater's Manifesto. Penguin Press.

Singh, S. (2006). "Impact of Color on Marketing." Management Decision.

The power of nostalgia and its role in making you purchase food

Gabriel, Y. (2019). Nostalgia: A Psychological Resource. Routledge.

Herz, R. (2016). Why You Eat What You Eat: The Science Behind Our Relationship with Food. Norton.

Holak, S. L., & Havlena, W. J. (1998). "Feelings, Fantasies, and Memories: An Examination of the Emotional Components of Nostalgia." Journal of Business Research.

Loveland, K. E., et al. (2010). "Nostalgia as a Resource for the Self." Self and Identity.

Routledge, C., et al. (2013). "The Power of the Past: Nostalgia as a Meaning-Making Resource." Memory.

How food claims work

Andrews, J. C., et al. (2014). *"Consumer Research on Front-of-Package Nutrition Ratings."*

References

EFSA. (2022). *"Guidance on Scientific Requirements for Health Claims."*

Grunert, K. G., & Wills, J. M. (2007). *"A Review of European Research on Consumer Response to Nutrition Information."*

Moss, M. (2013). *"Salt Sugar Fat: How the Food Giants Hooked Us."*

Schuldt, J. P., et al. (2012). *"The Organic Health Halo Effect."*

Branding for the sake of differentiation – Private label

Brandt, A. M. (2007). The cigarette century: The rise, fall, and deadly persistence of the product that defined America. Basic Books.

Dangour, A. D., et al. (2009). Nutritional quality of organic foods: A systematic review. American Journal of Clinical Nutrition, 90(3), 680–685. https://doi.org/10.3945/ajcn.2009.28041

Lustig, R. H. (2013). Fat chance: Beating the odds against sugar, processed food, obesity, and disease. Hudson Street Press.

Mozaffarian, D., et al. (2006). Trans fatty acids and cardiovascular disease. New England Journal of Medicine, 354(15), 1601–1613. https://doi.org/10.1056/NEJMra054035

Nestle, M. (2013). Food politics: How the food industry influences nutrition and health (Rev. ed.). University of California Press.

Scrinis, G. (2013). Nutritionism: The science and politics of dietary advice. Columbia University Press.

The issue with the word NATURAL

U.S. Food and Drug Administration (FDA). (2023). Use of the term "natural" in food labeling. Retrieved from https://www.fda.gov

European Food Safety Authority (EFSA). (2018). Scientific opinion on the definition of "natural" in food labeling. EFSA Journal, 16(12). [DOI:10.2903/j.efsa.2018.5487]

Nestle, M. (2018). Unsavory truth: How food companies skew the science of what we eat. Basic Books.

Lustig, R. H. (2020). Metabolical: The lure and the lies of processed food, nutrition, and modern medicine. Harper Wave.

Why natural, real, no nasties are meaningless words

European Food Safety Authority (EFSA). (2021). Food additives: Safety and regulation. https://www.efsa.europa.eu

References

U.S. Food and Drug Administration (FDA). (2023). Generally Recognized as Safe (GRAS) ingredients. https://www.fda.gov

Nestle, M. (2013). Food politics: How the food industry influences nutrition and health. University of California Press.

Warner, M. (2013). Pandora's lunchbox: How processed food took over the American meal. Scribner.

Stop being worried about the word CHEMICAL

Magnuson, B., et al. (2013). *Review of the regulation and safety assessment of food substances.* Regulatory Toxicology and Pharmacology, 65(1), 79-89.

Schwarcz, J. (2016). *Monkeys, Myths, and Molecules.* ECW Press.

Song, H., & Schwarz, N. (2009). *If it's hard to pronounce, it must be risky.* Psychological Science, 20(2), 135-138.

Shrinkflation: The art of distraction in food marketing

NielsenIQ. (2023). Global shrinkflation trends in FMCG. Retrieved from https://nielseniq.com

Wiggins, J. (2021). The psychology of packaging and consumer deception. Journal of Marketing Behavior, 6(2), 45-67. [DOI:10.1561/jm.2021.6.2]

Consumer Reports. (2023). How to spot shrinkflation at the grocery store. https://www.consumerreports.org

Convenience: More than just the packaging

Marsh, K., & Bugusu, B. (2007). Food packaging Roles, materials, and environmental issues. *Journal of Food Science, 72*(3), R39-R55. https://doi.org/10.1111/j.1750-3841.2007.00301.x

Robertson, G. L. (2016). *Food packaging: Principles and practice* (3rd ed.). CRC Press.

Verghese, K., Lewis, H., Lockrey, S., & Williams, H. (2015). Packaging's role in minimizing food loss and waste across the supply chain. *Packaging Technology and Science, 28*(7), 603-620. https://doi.org/10.1002/pts.2127

Wansink, B. (2016). *Slim by design: Mindless eating solutions for everyday life*. HarperCollins.

Price: Paying for convenience and quality

Aaker, D. A. (1996). Building strong brands. *Free Press.*

Hui, S. K., et al. (2013). Deconstructing the "first moment of truth." *Journal of Marketing Research, 50*(4), 445-463.

Lee, W. J., et al. (2013). How much will consumers pay for organic labels? *Journal of Consumer Research, 40*(4), 824-837.

References

Wansink, B. (2016). *Slim by design: Mindless eating solutions for everyday life*. HarperCollins.

Flavours

Burdock, G. A. (2016). *Fenaroli's handbook of flavor ingredients*. CRC Press.

FSANZ. (2023). *Standard 1.2.4 – Labelling of ingredients*. https://www.foodstandards.gov.au

NCCIH. (2019). *Artificial Food Colors and Attention-Deficit/Hyperactivity Symptoms*. https://www.nccih.nih.gov/health/artificial-food-colors-and-attention-deficithyperactivity-symptoms

Spence, C. (2015). *The science of flavour*. Oxford University Press.

The Daily Intake (DI)

Protein

Bauer, J., Biolo, G., Cederholm, T., Cesari, M., Cruz-Jentoft, A. J., Morley, J. E., … & Visvanathan, R. (2013). Evidence-based recommendations for optimal dietary protein intake in older people: A position paper from the PROT-AGE Study Group. *Journal of the American Medical Directors Association, 14*(8), 542–559. https://doi.org/10.1016/j.jamda.2013.05.021

Deer, R. R., & Volpi, E. (2015). Protein intake and muscle function in older adults. *Current Opinion in Clinical Nutrition & Metabolic Care, 18*(3), 248–253. https://doi.org/10.1097/MCO.0000000000000162

Jäger, R., Kerksick, C. M., Campbell, B. I., Cribb, P. J., Wells, S. D., Skwiat, T. M., … & Antonio, J. (2017). International Society of Sports Nutrition position stand: Protein and exercise. *Journal of the International Society of Sports Nutrition, 14*(1), 20. https://doi.org/10.1186/s12970-017-0177-8

Morton, R. W., Murphy, K. T., McKellar, S. R., Schoenfeld, B. J., Henselmans, M., Helms, E., … & Phillips, S. M. (2018). A systematic review, meta-analysis and meta-regression of the effect of protein supplementation on resistance training-induced gains in muscle mass and strength in healthy adults. *British Journal of Sports Medicine, 52*(6), 376–384. https://doi.org/10.1136/bjsports-2017-097608

National Health and Medical Research Council (NHMRC). (2013). *Australian dietary guidelines.* https://www.eatforhealth.gov.au

Volpi, E., Nazemi, R., & Fujita, S. (2013). Muscle tissue changes with aging. *Current Opinion in Clinical Nutrition & Metabolic Care, 7*(4), 405–410. https://doi.org/10.1097/01.mco.0000134362.76653.b2

References

Cruzat, V., Rogero, M. M., Keane, K. N., Curi, R., & Newsholme, P. (2018). Glutamine: Metabolism and immune function, supplementation and clinical translation. *Nutrients, 10*(11), 1564. https://doi.org/10.3390/nu10111564

Hou, Y., Wu, G., & Yin, Y. (2015). Functional amino acids in nutrition and health. *Amino Acids, 47*(1), 1-2. https://doi.org/10.1007/s00726-015-1956-7

National Health and Medical Research Council. (2013). *Nutrient reference values for Australia and New Zealand: Protein*. https://www.nrv.gov.au/nutrients/protein

Shimomura, Y., Yamamoto, Y., Bajotto, G., Sato, J., Murakami, T., Shimomura, N., … & Mawatari, K. (2006). Nutraceutical effects of branched-chain amino acids on skeletal muscle. *The Journal of Nutrition, 136*(2), 529S-532S. https://doi.org/10.1093/jn/136.2.529S

Whitney, E., Rolfes, S. R., Crowe, T., Cameron-Smith, D., & Walsh, A. (2017). *Understanding nutrition* (4th ed.). Cengage Learning Australia.

Fat

Australian Institute of Health and Welfare (AIHW). (2017). *A picture of overweight and obesity in Australia*. https://www.aihw.gov.au

DiNicolantonio, J. J., O'Keefe, J. H., & Lucan, S. C. (2016). Added fructose: A principal driver of type

2 diabetes mellitus and its consequences. *Mayo Clinic Proceedings, 90*(3), 372–381. https://doi.org/10.1016/j.mayocp.2014.12.019

Estruch, R., Ros, E., Salas-Salvadó, J., et al. (2013). Primary prevention of cardiovascular disease with a Mediterranean diet. *New England Journal of Medicine, 368*(14), 1279–1290. https://doi.org/10.1056/NEJMoa1200303

Harvard Health Publishing. (2020). *Oatmeal and cholesterol: A heart-healthy breakfast.* Harvard Medical School. https://www.health.harvard.edu/heart-health/oatmeal-and-cholesterol-a-heart-healthy-breakfast

Ludwig, D. S., Hu, F. B., Tappy, L., & Brand-Miller, J. (2018). Dietary carbohydrates: Role of quality and quantity in chronic disease. *BMJ, 361*, k2340. https://doi.org/10.1136/bmj.k2340

National Health and Medical Research Council (NHMRC). (2013). *Australian dietary guidelines.* https://www.eatforhealth.gov.au

Simopoulos, A. P. (2016). An increase in the omega-6/omega-3 fatty acid ratio increases the risk for obesity. *Nutrients, 8*(3), 128. https://doi.org/10.3390/nu8030128

Swanson, D., Block, R., & Mousa, S. A. (2012). Omega-3 fatty acids EPA and DHA: Health benefits throughout life. *Advances in Nutrition, 3*(1), 1–7. https://doi.org/10.3945/an.111.000893

References

Carbohydrates

Brand-Miller, J., et al. (2009). *Glycaemic index, postprandial glycaemia, and the shape of the curve.* Diabetes Care, 32(Suppl 2), S141–S146. https://doi.org/10.2337/dc09-S318

Jeukendrup, A. E. (2017). *Carbohydrate intake during exercise and performance.* Nutrition, 33, 1–8. https://doi.org/10.1016/j.nut.2016.06.004

Weickert, M. O., & Pfeiffer, A. F. (2018). *Impact of dietary fibre consumption on insulin resistance.* Diabetologia, 61(1), 1–13. https://doi.org/10.1007/s00125-017-4390-4

Slavin, J. (2013). *Fibre and prebiotics: Mechanisms and health benefits.* Nutrients, 5(4), 1417–1435. https://doi.org/10.3390/nu5041417

Becoming a Food Detective: Your Practical Toolkit – For Foods Sake!

Harris, J. L., Pomeranz, J. L., Lobstein, T., & Brownell, K. D. (2009). A crisis in the marketplace: How food marketing contributes to childhood obesity and what can be done. *Annual Review of Public Health, 30*, 211-225. https://doi.org/10.1146/annurev.publhealth.031308.100304

Monteiro, C. A., Cannon, G., Levy, R. B., Moubarac, J.-C., Jaime, P., Martins, A. P., Canella, D., Louzada,

M., & Parra, D. (2019). Ultra-processed foods: What they are and how to identify them. *Public Health Nutrition, 22*(5), 936–941. https://doi.org/10.1017/S1368980018003762

Moss, M. (2013). *Salt sugar fat: How the food giants hooked us*. Random House.

Moderation and Balance

Australian Bureau of Statistics. (2018). *National Health Survey: First results, 2017-18*. https://www.abs.gov.au/statistics/health/health-conditions-and-risks/national-health-survey-first-results/latest-release

Carabotti, M., Scirocco, A., Maselli, M. A., & Severi, C. (2015). The gut-brain axis: interactions between enteric microbiota, central and enteric nervous systems. *Annals of Gastroenterology*, *28*(2), 203–209.

Damasio, A. R. (1994). *Descartes' error: Emotion, reason, and the human brain*. Putnam.

Furman, D., Campisi, J., Verdin, E., Carrera-Bastos, P., Targ, S., Franceschi, C., … & Slavich, G. M. (2019). Chronic inflammation in the etiology of disease across the life span. *Nature Medicine*, *25*(12), 1822–1832. https://doi.org/10.1038/s41591-019-0675-0

Gearhardt, A. N., Yokum, S., Orr, P. T., Stice, E., Corbin, W. R., & Brownell, K. D. (2011). Neural correlates of food addiction. *Archives of General*

Psychiatry, 68(8), 808–816. https://doi.org/10.1001/archgenpsychiatry.2011.32

Mikkelsen, K., Stojanovska, L., Polenakovic, M., Bosevski, M., & Apostolopoulos, V. (2017). Exercise and mental health. *Maturitas, 106*, 48–56. https://doi.org/10.1016/j.maturitas.2017.09.003

Monteiro, C. A., Cannon, G., Levy, R. B., Moubarac, J.-C., Jaime, P., Martins, A. P., … & Parra, D. (2019). Ultra-processed foods: What they are and how to identify them. *Public Health Nutrition, 22*(5), 936–941. https://doi.org/10.1017/S1368980018003762

Nestle, M. (2013). *Food politics: How the food industry influences nutrition and health* (10th anniversary ed.). University of California Press.

Oliver, J. (2010). *Jamie's food revolution: Rediscover how to cook simple, delicious, affordable meals*. Hyperion.

World Health Organization. (2020). *WHO guidelines on physical activity and sedentary behaviour*. https://www.who.int/publications/i/item/9789240015128

What is improving in the food industry?

Australian Food and Grocery Council [AFGC]. (2022). *Sustainability Commitment Report*. https://afgc.org.au/sustainability/

CSIRO. (2021). *National Food Waste Strategy Feasibility Study*. https://www.csiro.au/en/research/natural-environment/biodiversity/food-waste

Food Standards Australia New Zealand [FSANZ]. (2023). *Health Star Rating system*. https://www.foodstandards.gov.au/consumer/labelling/Pages/Health-Star-Rating-system.aspx

Lawrence, M. et al. (2022). Food labelling and policy in Australia: Public health vs corporate power. *Public Health Nutrition*, *25*(8), 2128–2136. https://doi.org/10.1017/S1368980022001345

McClements, D. J. (2020). *Future Foods: How Modern Science Is Transforming the Way We Eat*. Springer Nature.

Monteiro, C. A. et al. (2019). Ultra-processed foods: What they are and how to identify them. *Public Health Nutrition*, *22*(5), 936–941. https://doi.org/10.1017/S1368980018003762

www.ingramcontent.com/pod-product-compliance
Lightning Source LLC
Chambersburg PA
CBHW041157280326
41927CB00019BA/3375